to Huda Mae
With best wishes for
a brilliant future

Don Richardson
1974

# THE PULVINAR-LP COMPLEX

# THE PULVINAR-LP COMPLEX

I. S. COOPER

M. RIKLAN

P. RAKIC

*Editors*

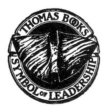

CHARLES C THOMAS • PUBLISHER

*Springfield • Illinois • U.S.A.*

*Published and Distributed Throughout the World by*

CHARLES C THOMAS • PUBLISHER

BANNERSTONE HOUSE

301–327 East Lawrence Avenue, Springfield, Illinois, U.S.A.

© *1974, by* CHARLES C THOMAS • PUBLISHER

ISBN 0-398-02849-4

Library of Congress Catalog Card Number: 73–15708

**Library of Congress Cataloging in Publication Data**

Main entry under title:

The Pulvinar-LP complex.

Papers presented at a symposium held at St. Barnabas Hospital, Bronx, N.Y.
1. Thalamus—Congresses. 1. Cooper, Irving Spencer, 1922- ed. II. Riklan, Manuel, ed. III. Rakic, P., ed. [DNLM: 1. Thalamus—Physiology—Congresses. WL312 P983 1972]
QP383.5.P84      612'.826      73–15708
ISBN O–398–02849–4

*Printed in the United States of America*

*BB-14*

# CONTRIBUTORS

I. AMIN, M.D.

*Department of Neurologic Surgery*
*St. Barnabas Hospital, Bronx, New York*

J. W. BROWN, M.D.

*Department of Neurology*
*St. Barnabas Hospital, Bronx, New York*

R. CHANDRA, M.D.

*Department of Neurologic Surgery*
*St. Barnabas Hospital, Bronx, New York*

I. S. COOPER, M.D., Ph.D.

*Department of Neurologic Surgery*
*St. Barnabas Hospital, Bronx, New York*

E. CRIGHEL, M.D.

*Department of Clinical and Experimental Neurophysiology*
*Institute of Neurology and Psychiatry, Bucharest, Rumania*

S. FASANO, M.D.

*University of Torino*
*Turin, Italy*

L. FRANKS, M.D.

*Department of Neurosurgery*
*Northwestern University Medical School, Chicago, Ill.*

T. L. FRIGYESI, M.D.

*Kantonspital, University of Zurich*
*Zurich, Switzerland*

S. GILMAN, M.D.

*Department of Neurology*
*Columbia University, New York, New York*

S. JACKSON, M.A.

*Speech and Hearing Department*
*St. Barnabas Hospital, Bronx, New York*

A. KREINDLER, M.D.

*Institute of Neurology and Psychiatry*
*Bucharest, Rumania*

G. A. OJEMANN, M.D.

*Department of Neurological Surgery*
*University of Washington, Seattle, Wash.*

L. POIRIER, M.D.

*Faculty of Medicine, Department of Medicine*
*Université Laval, Quebec, Canada*

P. RAKIC, M.D., Sc.D.

*Department of Neuropathology*
*Harvard Medical School, Boston, Mass.*

D. E. RICHARDSON, M.D.

*Department of Surgery, Division of Neurologic Surgery*
*Tulane University Medical School, New Orleans, Louisiana*

M. RIKLAN, Ph.D.

*Department of Psychology*
*St. Barnabas Hospital, Bronx, New York*

J. SIEGFRIED, M.D.

*Kantonspital, University of Zurich*
*Zurich, Switzerland*

E. B. SIQUEIRA, M.D.

*Neurosurgical Research Laboratory*
*Chicago Wesley Memorial Hospital, Chicago, Illinois*

M. TRACHTENBERG, Ph.D.

*Neuropsychology Laboratory*
*McLean Hospital, Belmont, Mass.*

J. VAN BUREN, M.D.

*National Institute of Neurological Diseases and Stroke*
*Bethesda, Maryland*

J. M. WALTZ, M.D.

*Department of Neurologic Surgery*
*St. Barnabas Hospital, Bronx, New York*

D. WEISSMAN, M.A.

*Department of Psychology*
*Fordham University, Bronx, New York*

# PREFACE

I SHOULD LIKE TO extend a sincere welcome to the partici-
pants in this symposium on behalf of my colleagues and myself. As you know, we have gathered here to explore an
unknown territory—the pulvinar, referred to by Walker, a
pioneer among thalamic explorers, as the terra incognita of
the thalamus. It is our aim to describe what is presently known
about the origin, structure and function of the pulvinar, or
LP-pulvinar complex, and to suggest possible avenues of fruit-
ful research for the future.

We can hope, at best, by bringing together what is presently
known about the pulvinar, to make a beginning into an eluci-
dation of its function in man, and of the possible therapeutic
usefulness of this information. By focusing our attention on
this somewhat unique structure, which appears to have
polysensory as well as motor functions, we may also be able
to contribute to a reconsideration of the functional role of
the entire thalamus; its nuclear classification, and the concept
of specific and non-specific nuclei.

Any one who has seriously pursued functional surgery of
the human brain, which is necessarily investigated and
studied under conditions of life, rather than under the experimental conditions of the biologic laboratory, must be constantly perplexed, confounded and stimulated by the seemingly capricious results and the paradoxes one encounters. It
has become evident that so-called specific relay nuclei, such as
the ventrolateral nucleus of the thalamus, also contribute considerably to so-called non-specific thalamo-cortical relations.
On the other hand, nuclei which had been categorized as
non-specific, such as centrum medianum, have been observed
clinically to play an important role in the physiology of such
diverse clinical phenomena as pain, chorea, and dystonia.
Consequently, consideration has been given to the desirabil-

ity of considering such nuclei as polysensory rather than as non-specific, and to redefining the precise role of the so-called relay nuclei.

Among the paradoxes which one encounters in functional surgery of the human thalamus are such observations as the fact that a lesion in the ventrolateral nucleus of the thalamus can abolish parkinsonian tremor or essential tremor or intentional tremor or rigidity from the contralateral limbs, if such symptoms exist. On the other hand, if a similar lesion is placed in a patient with torticollis, in whom no abnormality is observed in the extremities, no discernable change in motor or sensory function of the contralateral limbs can be elicited. Similarly, a lesion in centrum medianum in a patient with intractable pain may, in some instances, contribute to alleviation of the painful syndrome. A lesion in the same nucleus in a patient with dystonia musculorum deformans may, in some instances, contribute to an abolition of the dystonic symptoms. In contrast, even when such lesions are placed unilaterally or even bilaterally, specific neurologic deficits or electro-physiologic changes are usually not encountered. Consequently, this nucleus also may be more profitably investigated as a polysensory communication processor rather than as a non-specific structure.

The paradoxes which one encounters during a broad experience with physiologic surgery of the human thalamus include the observation that a lesion in one of the thalamic nuclei on one side of the cerebrum may produce a different effect than an identically placed lesion in the same nucleus in the opposite cerebral hemisphere in the same patient. In considering the apparently polysensory nature of virtually all of the nuclei of the thalamus, of the varying clinical effects observed following stimulation or lesioning of these nuclei under different physiologic and pathologic conditions, one is reminded of Snider's conclusion regarding the cerebellum: that it appears to function in direct response to the specific needs of the individual organism. Thus, what may seem at our present stage of knowledge to be capricious behavior of a neurologic structure, may actually be so sophisticated as to be beyond our present capabilities of evaluation.

In none of the regions of the thalamus does this statement seem to apply as directly as it does to the pulvinar. It is paradoxical in that its embryologic origin appears to arise at least, in part, from a telencephalic anlage quite different from that of the remainder of the thalamus. The effects of therapeutic lesions within the LP-pulvinar complex in humans have been observed to have a profound beneficial sensory and motor consequence in some patients, while in others with apparently similar syndromes the effect of a similar lesion has not been noteworthy. Although known to receive sensory input from virtually all of the sensory systems, it has been demonstrated both in the animal laboratory and in humans that large portions of this nuclear complex can be sacrificed without any observable neurologic or behavioral deficit.

I think that although we can state at the outset that the world will not long remember what we have gathered to say here, I do earnestly believe that our symposium will help to focus attention on this seemingly capricious but intriguing and obviously important neurologic structure. If we can accomplish that, can stimulate and cross fertilize each other in our varying disciplines and approaches to the study of the Pulvinar, and can have an interesting and enjoyable time here together, the purposes of this symposium will have been well served. I am certain that many more questions will be raised than answered. If that were not the case, the need for this symposium would not have arisen. I, for one, am pleased that the need has arisen and has provided my colleagues and myself here at St. Barnabas Hospital with the opportunity of welcoming you as contributors to this multidisciplinary investigation.

Irving S. Cooper, M.D., Ph.D.
March 8, 1972

# ACKNOWLEDGMENTS

W E ARE VERY pleased to acknowledge the collaboration and assistance of a number of individuals who participated at various stages in the planning, execution and publication of this symposium. First, appreciation is expressed to all of the individual contributors whose investigations formed the basis for this symposium. Gratitude is also expressed to the Board of Managers and Administration of St. Barnabas Hospital, particularly Mr. Charles M. Bliss, President of the Board of Managers, and Mr. John T. Kolody, Executive Director, for making available necessary hospital facilities. We are also grateful to Rose Marie Spitaleri and Lisa Cooper, photographers, and Mary Lorenc, medical artist, for their contributions during the symposium and in the publication of the manuscripts. We acknowledge also the efforts of Anne David, Juanit Newell, and Janet Dowling for their diligent and careful editing and typing of the various manuscripts. Finally, special thanks are offered to The John A. Hartford Foundation, Inc., New York City, for its many years of research support to the Department of Neurologic Surgery of St. Barnabas Hospital, including support for studies in pulvinectomy for hypertonicity.

# CONTENTS

# THE PULVINAR-LP
# COMPLEX

# CHAPTER 1

# EMBRYONIC DEVELOPMENT OF THE PULVINAR-LP COMPLEX IN MAN

P. Rakic, M.D., Sc.D

### I. Anatomical definition and phylogenetic development.

THE PULVINAR OCCUPIES the posterior pole of the ovoid-shaped human thalamus. Its large caudal extension, covered with pia, overhangs the geniculate bodies and superior colliculus. The entire volume of the pulvinar consists of lightly stained multipolar neurons of medium and small sizes, distributed among numerous fibers that demarcate it rather clearly from most of the adjacent thalamic components. Cellular constellations within the nucleus itself permit a somewhat arbitrary subdivision of the pulvinar into medial, lateral, and inferior portions. The nucleus lateralis posterior (LP) is situated in front of the pulvinar bounded by the nucleus ventralis lateralis, nucleus ventralis posterior, nucleus centrum medianum, and nucleus medialis dorsalis. A similar cellular composition of the LP and pulvinar makes the borderline between these two thalamic components rather vague, and has led to use of the term "LP-pulvinar complex."

The pulvinar is phylogenetically the most recent nucleus of the dorsal thalamus. Rodents lack this thalamic component. It appears as a relatively small but rather clearly outlined nucleus in carnivores increasing progressively in size from monkeys to apes, until in man it reaches enormous proportions (see references in Rakic and Sidman, 1969). It is, therefore, not surprising that the impetus for this Symposium devoted

3

to the LP-pulvinar complex has come from those concerned with the human brain.

Since the pulvinar in man is the largest thalamic nucleus, it is remarkable that we know so little about its connections and functions. The generally accepted hypothesis that the pulvinar and the adjacent LP nucleus play a crucial role in the sensory integrative mechanism of the thalamus was based on its progressive evolutionary development in relation to other thalamic components and its reciprocal connections with parieto-temporo-occipital neocortex, rather than on clear-cut physiological or clinical data. The increasing size of the pulvinar during phylogenesis occurs *pari-passu* with the expansion and elaboration of the homotypical neocortex of the parieto-temporo-occipital areas. It has been speculated that phyletic elaboration of these thalamic and cerebral structures as a unit might be related to the increasingly complex behavioral response to the environment in primates (e.g., Smith, 1910; Yakovlev, 1969; Geschwind, 1965). Indeed, the so-called "association" neocortex to which the pulvinar projects is strategically situated at the borders of three major sensory areas, somesthetic, visual and auditory. Different portions of the pulvinar and LP in the cat seem to project to specific regions of this cortex (Graybiel, 1972 a,b) but hodological details in man remain to be discovered. Knowledge of the afferent input to the LP-pulvinar complex is even more scanty. The study of serially sectioned human brains with focal cortical or thalamic lesions (e.g., Van Buren, this symposium) provides the most valuable information but unfortunately with no control of the distribution or timing of the lesions.

This report deals with the embryological development of the LP-pulvinar complex in man. The data are based mostly on material published with more complete documentation elsewhere (Rakic and Sidman, 1969). In addition, I shall consider some more general notions about the dual origin of pulvinar neurons and the possible relationship between development of the pulvinar and histogenesis of those areas of the cerebral neocortex to which it projects.

## II. CELL BEHAVIOR DURING EARLY DEVELOPMENT OF THE THALAMUS

At the end of the 4th embryonic week, almost the full thickness of the diencephalic wall is composed of a ventricular zone,[1] with only an incipient marginal zone present externally (fig. 1A). The ventricular zone is composed of uniformly distributed, densely packed, darkly stained proliferative cells with numerous mitotic figures at the ventricular surface. The

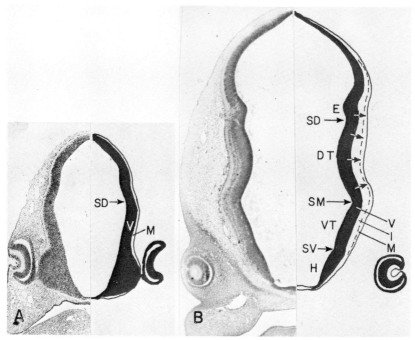

Figure 1–1. A. Microphotograph (left half) and outline drawing (right half) of a transverse section through the diencephalon of an approximately 4-week human fetus. The entire neural wall consists of ventricular (V) and marginal (M) zones. The sulcus dorsalis (SD) is just discernible.

B. Diencephalon of an approximately 6-week human fetus. The neural wall consists by now of ventricular (V), intermediate (I) and marginal (M) zones. Sulcus ventralis (SV), medius (SM), and dorsalis (SD) clearly demarcate major diencephalic components, the hypothalamus (H), ventral thalamus (VT), dorsal thalamus (DT), and epithalamus (E), respectively.

---

[1] Nomenclature recommendations of the Boulder Committee, *Anat. Rec. 166* 257–262, 1970, have been adopted.

cell-sparse marginal zone consists of outward-directed processes of ventricular cells. As some cells become permanently
postmitotic their cell bodies move out of the proliferative
layer and form a new band, the intermediate zone, interposed
between the ventricular and marginal zones (fig. 1B). The
intermediate zone is distinguished by its larger, rounder, and
more widely spaced nuclei compared to the predecessor nuclei in the ventricular zone. Autoradiographic analysis of histogenesis of the mouse thalamus (Angevine, 1970a) confirmed
that cells of the ventricular zone undergo their last division
close to the ventricular surface and then move to the intermediate zone. Concomitantly, the medial (ventricular) surface
of the diencephalic wall develops three shallow longitudinal
grooves: sulcus dorsalis, medius and ventralis (Herrick, 1910),
which delineate the prospective epithalamus, dorsal
thalamus, ventral thalamus and hypothalamus (fig. 1B). Thus
by the 6th fetal week the human diencephalic wall in the
region of prospective thalamus consists of three fundamental
embryonal zones and contains numerous postmitotic neurons
which have arisen at the ventricular surface.

Histological studies of thalamic development in different
animals (Miura, 1933; Rose, 1942; Niimi, Harada, Kuska and
Kishi, 1962) and the autoradiographic analysis of the time
of cell origin in the mouse thalamus (Angevine, 1970a) can
be correlated with the early developmental events in the
human diencephalon (Gilbert, 1935; Dekaban, 1954; Kahle,
1956). In the mouse, almost all thalamic neurons are generated
in the ventricular zone during a relatively early and brief
span of time (Angevine, 1970a). The positions of neuron somas
in the adult mouse thalamus reflect a three-dimensional
gradient system with respect to time of neuron origin. The
gradients, from earliest-generated to latest-generated cells,
follow ventral-dorsal, lateral-medial, and caudal-rostral vec-
tors. These gradients are smooth and appear to ignore the
anatomist's histoarchitectonic subdivisions of the organ into
discrete nuclei. Presumably the gradients reflect corresponding spatial and temporal gradients in the thalamic ventricular
zone during the embryonic period of neuron genesis (Angevine, 1970a).

In man by the 8th week the ventricular zone of the diencephalon has become considerably wider in the region of the prospective dorsal thalamus (fig. 2). It produces new waves of postmitotic neurons continually for several weeks before fading out in the 13th to 15th fetal weeks (Dekaban, 1954; Rakic and Sidman, 1969).

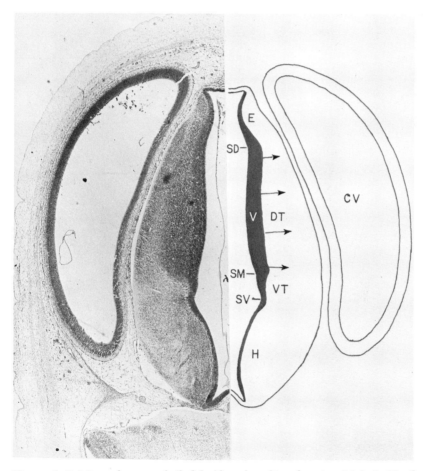

Figure 1–2. Microphotograph (left half) and outline drawing (right half) of a transverse section through the diencephalon of an 8-week human fetus. Abbreviations are the same as in figure 1 with addition of CV, cerebral vesicle.

## III. CYTOARCHITECTONIC DIFFERENTIATION OF THE THALAMIC NUCLEI

During the period of proliferative activity described above, the diencephalic wall in the region of the prospective thalamus increases several times in thickness (fig. 4) and all thalamic nuclei gradually become discernable cytoarchitectonically. Subdivision of the thalamus into discrete nuclear groups appears to be based initially on the establishment of boundaries by fascicles of nerve fibers. Only later do the nuclear groups acquire individuality in terms of cell soma size, shape, and staining intensity as seen in Nissl images.

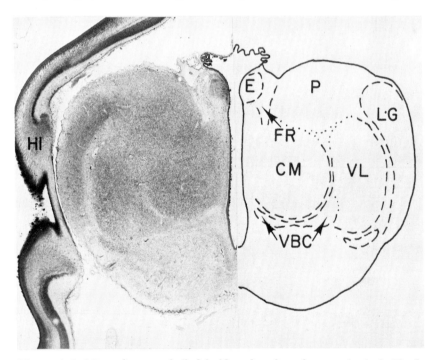

Figure 1–3. Microphotograph (left half) and outline drawing (right half) of a coronal section through the posterior part of the thalamus of a 13-week human fetus. The boundaries of various thalamic nuclei are recognized by the cell-sparse bordering zones between them, even though the young neurons look alike in all thalamic nuclei at these stages.

Abbreviations: CM, nucleus centrum medianum; E, epithalamus; FR, fasciculus retroflexus; HI, hippocampus; LG, lateral geniculate body; P, pulvinar; VBC, ventrobasal complex; VL, nucleus ventralis lateralis.

By the end of the 3rd month of gestation in man, fiber systems demarcate most of the ventral and posteroventral thalamic nuclei (fig. 3). The lateral (LG) and medial geniculate bodies, ventrobasal complex (VCB, with arrows indicating posterolateral and posteromedial divisions), nucleus centrum medianum (CM), and nucleus ventralis lateralis (VL) are well delineated. The medial dorsal nucleus emerges into view a bit more slowly and still appears continuous posteriorly with the common anlage of LP and the pulvinar (P). At this early stage the pulvinar and LP appear to be uniform in histological structure and represent simply the posterior thalamus. It is worth emphasizing that at this fetal age, the combined volume of both structures is smaller than the volume of the nucleus centrum medianum (compare P and CM in fig. 3). In adult, however, the pulvinar alone is several times larger than the centrum medianum.

## IV. THE DEVELOPMENT OF THE POSTERIOR GROUP OF THALAMIC NUCLEI

As illustrated in figures 3 and 4, at 13–15 fetal weeks the posterior part of the thalamus (P) has a proportionately small size relative to other thalamic nuclei. Indeed, at this stage of human brain development the positions of diencephalic components correspond approximately to their adult positions in subprimate species. The posterior portion of the human thalamus begins its extraordinary growth only after the 15th week, as demonstrated vividly in sagittal sections (fig. 5). The late growth of the pulvinar is demonstrable both by its continually increasing volume and by the prominent bulging of its dorsal and posterior portion into the transverse cerebral fissure. A direct outcome of the late development of the LP-pulvinar complex is the transformation of the human thalamus into a structure very different from that of most subprimate species. The massive pulvinar not only dominates the posterior part of the thalamus in man (figs. 4,5), but causes the lateral geniculate body to become gradually displaced ventrally from its initially dorsal position (fig. 4). In most non-

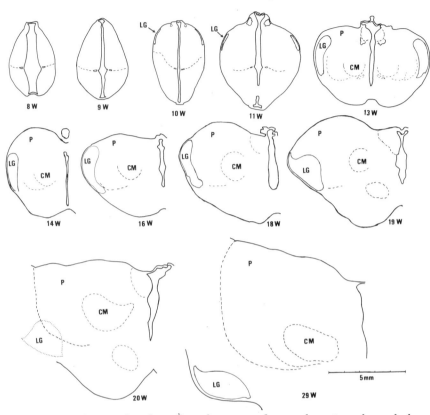

Figure 1–4. Camera lucida outline drawings of coronal sections through the diencephalon in human fetuses of 8 to 29 weeks of gestation. From Rakic and Sidman (1969). The pulvinar region (P) enlarges considerably after 16 weeks and gradually displaces the lateral geniculate body (LG) in a ventral and posterior direction. The nucleus centrum medianum (CM) is outlined as a reference point. All drawings are at the same magnification, as indicated by the scale at the lower right.

primate adult species which lack such pulvinar growth, the geniculate retains a dorsal position to adulthood (Clark, 1932).

Histoarchitectonically the pulvinar is the last nuclear mass in the entire diencephalon to acquire individuality. Its neurons show a protracted tempo of differentiation and myelin appears late (Yakovlev, 1969). The volume of individual neurons, number and size of glial cells, ingrowth of afferent axons, and establishment of vascular supply all contribute to the thalamic growth but these elements do not increase

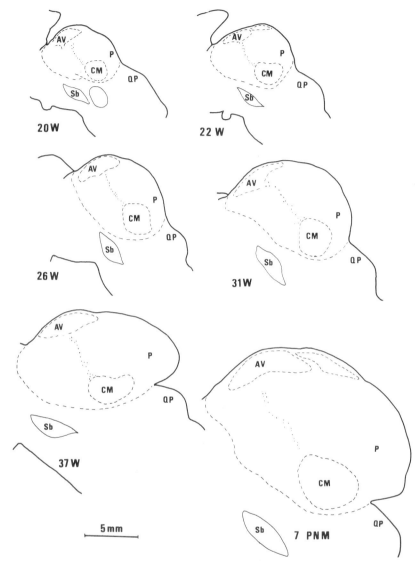

Figure 1–5. Camera lucida outline drawings of sagittal sections through the diencephalon in human fetuses of 20 weeks gestation (20 W) to 7 postnatal months (7 PNM). From Rakic and Sidman (1969). The individual figures are positioned so that a line from the anterior ventral nucleus (AV) to the centrum medianum (CM) always lies in the same orientation. The late growth of the pulvinar (P) is indicated by its continually increasing area and by the prominent bulging of its dorsal and posterior surfaces. The subthalamic nucleus (Sb) of the ventral thalamus and the quadrigeminal plate (QP) of the midbrain serve as reference points. The magnification is the same for all drawings as indicated by the scale at the lower left.

more rapidly in the pulvinar region than in other thalamic nuclei (e.g., Yakovlev, 1969). Therefore, it is reasonable to assume that the number of neurons in the pulvinar must continue to increase significantly during the middle trimester of human fetal development, when most of the other thalamic nuclei already have a full complement of neurons (Rakic and Sidman, 1969).

In the light of the late appearance of the pulvinar in phylogeny its relatively late onset and protracted span of embryologic development is not itself surprising. The puzzling fact is that the proliferative capacity of the ventricular zone of the diencephalon is already exhausted and has ceased to produce new neurons during the middle trimester when the pulvinar is undergoing its major growth. During this late period the ventricular surface of the 3rd ventricle consists of several well defined rows of cuboid cells with virtually no mitotic figures (Dekaban, 1954; Rakic and Sidman, 1969). Autoradiographic analysis of fragments of human thalamic tissue incubated supravitally in tritiated thymidine solutions has confirmed that the ventricular zone of the diencephalon at 18 and 22 fetal weeks no longer produces substantial number of cells (fig. 6A, and Rakic and Sidman, 1968, 1969).

## V. THE SOURCE OF LATE FORMING NEURONS FOR THE POSTERIOR THALAMUS

The only significant germinal epithelium in the general vicinity of the thalamus during late stages of pulvinar development lies across the sulcus terminalis in the floor of the lateral ventricle of the telencephalon, the so-called ganglionic eminence (figs. 7,8). In the same autoradiographic study mentioned in the previous paragraph, approximately 30 percent of the cells in small fragments cut from the ganglionic eminence of 18 and 22 week human fetuses were labeled after one hour of supravital incubation (fig. 6B). The ganglionic eminence can be viewed as an enormously expanded subventricular germinative zone of the telencephalon persisting throughout the fetal period in the floor of the lateral ventricles

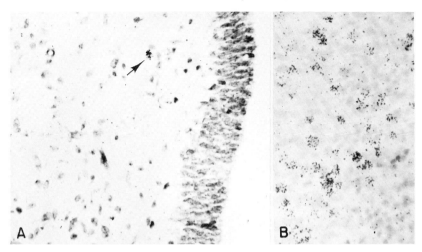

Figure 1–6. A. Autoradiogram of the thalamic surface adjacent to the third ventricle of an 18.5-week human fetus. The tissue was immersed supravitally in a tissue culture medium containing thymidine-$H^3$ for 1 hour. The ependyma forms a sharply demarcated, densely packed cellular zone, about 4 nuclei wide and contains no labeled cells. A few randomly positioned, well-labeled small round nuclei (arrow) deeper in the thalamus are interpreted as glia which proliferate *in situ*. For further details, see Rakic and Sidman (1968).
B. Autoradiogram of ganglionic eminence of the same fetus represented in figure 6A. The large number of labeled cells indicates high proliferative activity in this region.

(Rakic and Sidman, 1968, 1969; Boulder Committee, 1970). It consists of uniformly distributed, densely packed, darkly stained, undifferentiated germinal cells. The entire structure was considered by most investigators simply as the anlage of the basal ganglia, particularly of the adjacent caudate nucleus (e.g., Hamilton, Boyd and Mossman, 1952; Patten, 1953). Indeed, the caudate with its larger, lightly stained cells is almost completely surrounded by ganglionic eminence (figs. 7,8). However, the ganglionic eminence is disproportionately large in comparison to the caudate nucleus, as is particularly explicit in sagittal sections (fig. 8), and it has been suggested recently that this proliferative epithelium may contribute cells to a wider range of telencephalic and diencephalic structures (Rakic and Sidman, 1969; Karten, 1970).

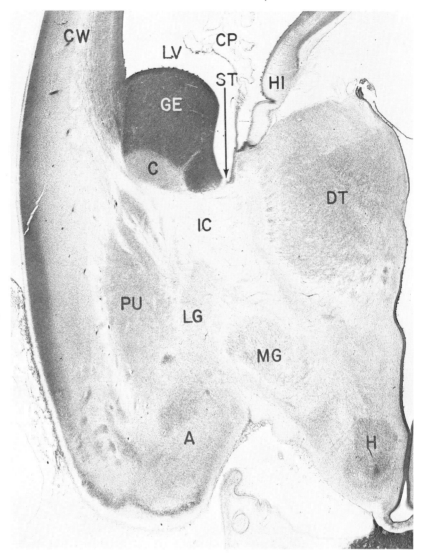

Figure 1–7. Coronal section through the di-telencephalic junction of a 12-week human fetus. The ganglionic eminence (GE) forms a thick bed of germinal cells above the anlage of the caudate nucleus (C) in the floor of the lateral ventricle (LV) and appears sharply separated from the dorsal thalamus (DT) at the sulcus terminalis (ST). Other abbreviations: A, amygdala; CP, choroid plexus; CW, cerebral wall; H, hypothalamus; HI, hippocampus; LG, lateral segment of the globus pallidus; MG, medial segment of the globus pallidus; PU, putamen.

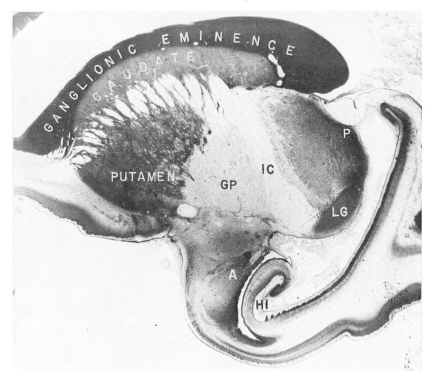

Figure 1–8. Sagittal section through the brain of a 22-week human fetus to illustrate the relationship between caudate, putamen, globus pallidus (GP) amygdala (A) and pulvinar (P) with the ganglionic eminence. This plane of section shows to advantage the size of the ganglionic eminence and its extent into the rostral-caudal axis, but leaves out the postero-inferior part except for the portion coating the amygdala (asterisk). Other abbreviations: IC, internal capsule; HI, hippocampus; LG, lateral geniculate body.

The ganglionic eminence would seem at first glance to be a rather unlikely candidate as a source of thalamic neurons, since at the time the migration should occur, it is already separated from the diencephalon by the relatively deep sulcus terminalis (fig. 7). However, in younger embryos this separation is by no means sharp. At somite stages of embryonic development, the prospective diencephalon and telencephalon are in continuity in the longitudinal axis and it is impossible to designate a di-telencephalic boundary that would provide a real embryological basis for a sharp distinction between these two formations (Källén, 1951). Éven in slightly older embryos (6 weeks) the rostro-lateral border of the thalamus is in continuity across the foramen of Monro with the ganglionic eminence, though by then a shallow sulcus terminalis has become discernable (fig. 9A). This sulcus constituting the di-telencephalic junction, shifts gradually posterolaterally and becomes deeper and more elongated as it is displaced caudally (fig. 9B,C). In this way, the original rostral and dorsal portion of the thalamus shifts during development to a lateral and posterior position (Hochstetter, 1919). Thus, the posterior thalamic region becomes separated from the ganglionic eminence only secondarily by a relatively deep sulcus terminalis (fig. 9C).

In spite of the separation by the sulcus terminalis, some cells seem to pass from the ganglionic eminence of the telencephalon into what is now the lateral and posterior parts of the diencephalon continuously during the period from 16 to 34 fetal weeks (Rakic and Sidman, 1969). Examination of more than 50 human fetal brains sectioned serially in the

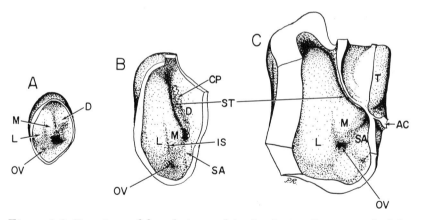

Figure 1–9. Drawings of dorsal views of the forebrain after removal of the neopallial dome to expose the floor of the hemispheric vesicle containing the lateral (L) and medial (M) ridges of the ganglionic eminence. Modified from Frazer (1940). Approximate fetal ages: A, 6 weeks; B, 8 weeks; C, 12 weeks. Abbreviations: AC, anterior commissure; CP, choroid plexus; D, diencephalon; IS, interstitial sulcus; L, lateral ridge of the ganglionic eminence; M, medial ridge of the ganglionic eminence; OV, olfactory ventricle; SA, septal area; ST, sulcus terminalis; T, thalamus dorsalis.

horizontal plane (approximately parallel to the plane passing through the anterior and posterior commissures) demonstrates the possible migratory pathways much better than the routinely used coronal plane. Two possible routes are indicated by arrows in the right hand drawing of fig. 10. The

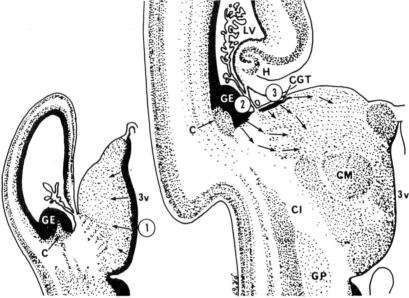

Figure 1–10. Semidiagrammatic drawings of the thalamus and adjacent parts of the cerebrum, sectioned in the horizontal plane. From Rakic and Sidman (1969). The arrows indicate the main paths of cell migration during formation of the thalamus. The left illustration is from a 10-week fetus at a magnification of about 8×. The right drawing is from a 24-week fetus at about 4×. The arrows near the circled number 1 indicate that the ventricular zone in the wall of the third ventricle serves as the source of thalamic neurons during early development. The arrows extending from the circled number 2 indicate the path of migration of cells from their origin in the ganglionic eminence (GE) across the incipient posterior thalamic peduncle and internal capsule to reach the lateral thalamus. The arrows at circled number 3 indicate another migration path that lies posterolaterally, the cells passing through the corpus gangliothalamicum (CGT) into the thalamus. Migrations 2 and 3 come at a stage when the ventricular zone of the third ventricle is exhausted and yet the lateral and superior parts of the thalamus are still expanding enormously. Other abbreviations: C, caudate nucleus; CI, internal capsule; CM, nucleus centrum medianum; GP, globus pallidus; H, hippocampal formation; LV, lateral ventricle; 3V, third ventricle.

first, rather speculative, is across the developing internal capsule and posterior thalamic radiation. The second route, based
on Nissl and Golgi evidence, follows a more superficial course
just beneath the sulcus terminalis and into the pulvinar region.
Undifferentiated cells were found to form a thin sheet approximately 200 $\mu$ wide and 2000 $\mu$ long which coats the caudalmost protuberance of the thalamus and is separated from the
pia by a marginal zone that is almost free of cells (fig. 11A).
The sheet consists of four to six layers of small undifferentiated cells with staining properties similar to cells in
the ganglionic eminence. This embryonic structure was interpreted as consisting of constantly changing populations migrating during the period from 18 to 34 weeks, and was named
the corpus gangliothalamicum according to the presumed
origin and terminus of the migrating cells (Rakic and Sidman,
1969). Both the behavior of the cells and the name are analogous to the transient migratory cell population of the embryonic
corpus pontobulbare of the brainstem described by Essick
(1912). In both cases the migrating cells occupy predomi-
nantly a superficial position and individual cells display a
bipolar shape, with their processes parallel to the surface
and elongated in the direction of migration (fig. 11B).

## VI. SOME SPECULATIONS CONCERNING
## EMBRYOLOGICAL DEVELOPMENT
## OF THE LP-PULVINAR COMPLEX

Several important unsolved problems related to the histogenesis of the posterior thalamus require separate consideration. (a) What percentage of pulvinar and LP cells are
formed at early stages from the ventricular and subventricular
zones of the third ventricle (left drawing in fig. 10) compared
to late forming cells of telencephalic origin (right drawing
in fig. 10)? (b) Do cells of these different origins belong to
morphologically or physiologically distinct classes in the adult
thalamus? (c) Are cells of telencephalic origin confined to
the pulvinar and LP nucleus or do some spill over to the
other thalamic components? The autoradiographic method
has not resolved these questions since the LP-pulvinar complex hardly exists in commonly used laboratory species (e.g.,

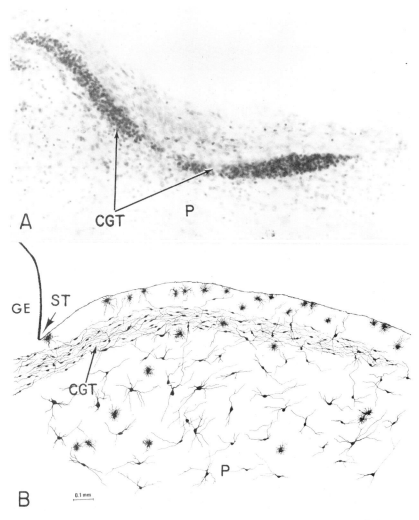

Figure 1–11. A. Corpus gangliothalamicum (CGT) of an 18-week human fetus. It consists of a sheet of densely packed undifferentiated cells situated at the posterior pulvinar surface (P).

B. Drawing of a Golgi preparation of the posterior thalamus, including a portion of the ganglionic eminence (GE), to indicate the position of cells and the gradient of their shapes from bipolar migrating cell close to the ganglionic eminence, to multipolar young neuron deeper in the thalamus. Other abbreviations: CGT, corpus gangliothalamicum, ST, sulcus terminalis. From Rakic and Sidman (1969). See text for further details. The scale at the bottom indicates the magnification.

Angevine, 1970a), and only now is being applied for the first time in the primate in work now in progress in our laboratory (e.g., Rakic, 1973a). At this moment the discussion must be presented in a somewhat speculative vein.

(a)  A significant portion of both pulvinar and LP are definitively formed before the corpus gangliothalamicum appears in human fetuses (fig. 3). Therefore, the cells which initially compose the anlage of pulvinar-LP complex most probably originate exclusively at the ventricular and subventricular zones lining the 3rd ventricle (fig. 10A). However, the absolute number of these early formed cells cannot be even approximated since the volume of LP-pulvinar complex at that age, the cell sizes and the rate of cell growth are completely unknown. An estimate of the relative number of late forming cells of telencephalic origin is similarly imprecise. It is, however, safe to state that in spite of its relatively small size, the corpus gangliothalamicum could theoretically supply a sizeable number of cells since it has prolonged existence of over four months (Rakic and Sidman, 1969). If cells in man migrate a distance of 2 mm a day, the rate estimated in the mouse corpus pontobulbare (Taber-Pierce, 1966; 1967); the total number of cells passing from telencephalon to diencephalon would be very high indeed.

(b)  The cell migration from the ganglionic eminence might represent simply a mechanism to supply the posterior thalamus in man with a larger number of undifferentiated and uncommitted neuron precursors, or alternatively, these late-forming cells might represent cells already committed to a particular neuron class. This remains to be worked out. However, numerous autoradiographic studies of the other components of the central nervous system have shown that different classes of neurons are usually generated on precise schedules (Angevine, 1970b; Sidman, 1970). For example, in the retina, cerebral and cerebellar cortices, hippocampus, pons, and olfactory bulb, most of the larger efferent neurons are generated first, followed by the smaller short axon, Golgi type II interneurons (Sidman, 1961; Miale and Sidman, 1961; Angevine, 1965; Altman, 1966; Hinds, 1968; Sidman, 1970). By analogy with the development of other brain structures, it seems reasonable to assume that late-forming neurons of telencephalic origin also give a rise to relatively small-sized interneurons, rather than to larger neurons that send their axons to distant sites. Though small thalamic neurons (microneurons) were already described in 1895 by Monakow (*spindelförmige Zellen und Schaltzellen*), few authors have dealt with them (Hassler, 1955; McLardy, 1963). They were considered to be the interneurons of the thalamus, and are found to be significantly more numerous in the association nuclei, particularly LP and pulvinar (Dewulf, 1971). The recent finding of a population of small thalamic neurons 3–5 $\mu$ in diameter, somewhat reminiscent of the cerebellar granule cells (Scheibel and Scheibel, 1972), is also rather intriguing. The significance of these cells, their distribution and ultrastructural identity is still unknown, and they have not been yet studied in primates, but the possible analogy with late forming cerebellar granule cells is too obvious to be overlooked. The only evidence that larger neurons of the pulvinar are indeed generated earlier than small ones comes from the observation that many of the larger cells already show a rather high degree of differentiation at the time when new cells migrate from the ganglionic eminence. These earlier-generated cells display a relatively large pale nucleus and well-developed Nissl granules (fig. 12A).

Some immature synaptic junctions are clearly in electron-micrographs of the pulvinar in the 22-week human fetus in spite of inadequate fixation of postmortem human tissue (fig. 12B,C). Therefore, in the pulvinar newly arrived neurons have to penetrate neuropil already interconnected with synaptic junctions. In this respect cells migrating to the pulvinar resemble cerebellar granule cells, which originate at late developmental stages in the external granular layer and subsequently traverse the molecular layer and the row of Purkinje cells that had been generated much earlier in the ventricular zone of the fourth ventricle (Ramón y Cajal, 1960; Miale and Sidman, 1961). Like cells from the corpus gangliothalamicum, granule cells during their migration penetrate a neuropil

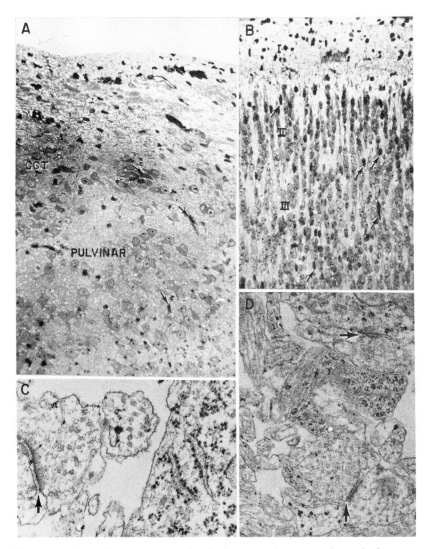

Figure 1–12. A. Photomicrograph of a horizontal section through the posterior pulvinar in a 22-week human fetus including medialmost portion
of the corpus gangliothalamicum (CGT). The arrows indicate the undifferentiated bipolar cells situated among larger cells with pale nuclei. The
specimen was embedded in EPON, sectioned at $1\,\mu$ and stained with
alkaline toluidine blue.
B. Microphotograph of the parietal neocortex (layers I-III) of the same
fetus. The tissue was prepared identically as in A. Arrows indicate undifferentiated bipolar cells on their way to superficial positions in the cortex.
C and D. Electron microscopic images of immature synapses in the pulvinar
of a 22-week human fetus.

which already contains numerous synaptic junctions (Rakic, 1971). Another similar example is seen during the late migration of cells from the rhombic lip over the lateral surface of the medulla and pons to form the inferior olive and nuclei griseum pontis (Essick, 1912; Taber-Pierce, 1966). Electron-microscopic analysis of this population of migrating cells in the rhesus monkey shows that many of them become intercalated in a neuropil already rich in synaptic connections (Rakic, unpublished). It seems that some brain structures require a greater number of neurons for their circuitry than was initially supplied from the ventricular zone. The mechanical problem of populating a region in which neurons are already interconnected may be easier if the new cells enter across a free external surface rather than directly through a complex neuropil. The genesis of the pulvinar, therefore, does not represent a unique case in the developing mammalian central nervous system.

One important qualification must be made concerning the designation of all cells which migrate from the ganglionic eminence into the posterior thalamus as exclusively neurons. The Golgi evidence of transitional forms from bipolar migrating cells to a typical multipolar shape indicates that many of the cells entering by 22 weeks are neurons. However, it is probable that, particularly at later stages, some cells might be glial precursors or uncommitted subventricular cells still able to transform into both neurons and glial cells (Schaper, 1897; Boulder Committee, 1970).

(c) The LP-pulvinar complex was considered the main recipient of cells of telencephalic origin primarily because of the close spatial relationship between the posterior thalamus and the ganglionic eminence and also because the corpus gangliothalamicum is situated in the caudalmost portion of the thalamus (Rakic and Sidman, 1969). This hypothesis was supported by the demonstration of transitional forms of neurons from a simple bipolar phase within the corpus gangliothalamicum itself to a multipolar stage found deeper in the pulvinar. However, the possibility was not ruled out that other thalamic components, particularly intralaminar

nuclei or association nuclei such as the parvocellular portion
of the nucleus medialis dorsalis, might also receive a certain
number of cells of telencephalic origin.

## VII. DEVELOPMENT OF RELATIONSHIP BETWEEN LP-PULVINAR COMPLEX AND THE NEOCORTEX

Several lines of evidence indicate that afferent fibers which
originate in the thalamus reach the cerebrum virtually at the
very beginning of the histogenesis of the cortical plate
(Poliakov, 1961; Yakovlev, 1969; Angevine, 1970a; Morest,
1970; Marin-Padilla, 1971). In man, the maturation of thalamic
neurons and the development of the thalamocortical projections anticipate by a week the development of homotypical
cortex (Yakovlev, 1969). The use of more specific methods
to assess the presence of fibers indicates that afferents may
be formed even much earlier than indicated by routine stains
(e.g., Windle, 1970). Among earliest cortical regions to appear
and the first to show signs of cytoarchitectonic maturation
are the specific projection areas which receive direct, com-
pact, precisely patterned inputs from the corresponding
thalamic nuclei. The cortical areas connected with the late-
forming thalamic nuclei themselves emerge considerably
later and have a prolonged developmental period. Thus,
thalamocortical projections may influence the tempo of maturation and relative size of different areas of the cerebral cortex.
Since the sequence of development and maturation of different thalamocortical projections was found to proceed in parallel both in phylogeny and ontogeny, it has been suggested
that development of the thalamus in some way determines
the size and organization of the specialized cortical areas (e.g.,
Smith, 1910). Indeed, the peculiarly human regions of parieto-
temporo-occipital neocortex begin to differentiate at later ages
than any other cerebral region according both to cytoarchitectonic (Poliakov, 1965) and myeloarchitectonic criteria
(Flechsig, 1920; Yakovlev and Lecours, 1967). The late
development and protracted cycle of differentiation of this
cortical territory correlates rather well with the late and protracted genesis of neuron somas of the pulvinar-LP complex,
which form its major source of afferents. It is most probable

that the basic thalamocortical projections are formed by neurons which have originated in the ventricular zone of the diencephalon. However, it would be important to know whether at later stages the single fountainhead, ganglionic eminence produces simultaneously young neurons destined to migrate into these two distant but synaptically related regions of diencephalon and telencephalon (fig. 13). It should be underscored that the migratory pathways from ganglionic eminence to the cortex marked by lines and arrows in fig. 13 represent only a speculative working hypothesis. Indeed, so far the only evidence we have is that a number of undif-

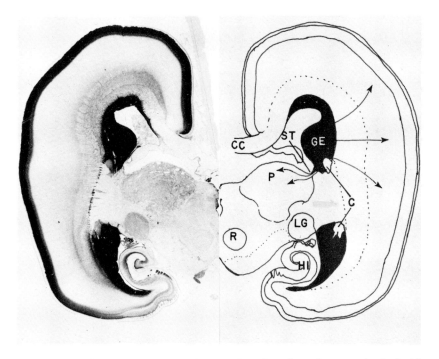

Figure 1–13. Photomicrograph (left half) and outline drawing (right half) of a coronal section through the brain of a 22-week human fetus to show the superior and inferior portions of the curving ganglionic eminence. Arrows indicate hypothetical migratory pathways for cells originating from a common portion of the ganglionic eminence. Further explanation in text. Abbreviations: CG, corpus callosum; GE, ganglionic eminence; HI, hippocampus; LG, lateral geniculate body; P, pulvinar; R, red nucleus; ST, sulcus terminalis.

ferentiated cells do migrate into the superficial layers of the neocortex (fig. 12B) during the period when the pulvinar is receiving from the ganglionic eminence cells of very similar morphology (fig. 12A). It is generally accepted that most of the late-forming cells of the neocortex differentiate into stellate cells (Golgi type II neurons) of the more superficial cortical layers and that these elements are phylogenetically the youngest neurons (Poliakov, 1965). However, the actual time and place of origin of this late-forming population has not been determined in man. The study of cell migration to the superficial layers of fetal monkey neocortex (Rakic, 1972) indicates that many late-forming cells are generated around the midgestational period in the subventricular zone. We expect that more detailed and precise information concerning development of the primate cortex, based on an autoradiographic analysis in rhesus monkey now under way in our laboratory will provide a direct test of these speculations.

## VIII. CONCLUSION

The pulvinar, the large posterior component of the thalamus, attains prominence in primates, particularly in man. Its phylogenetic development occurs concomitantly with the elaboration of the parieto-temporo-occipital neocortex with which it makes an anatomico-physiological unit. Embryologically in man it develops mostly in the middle trimester, after the basic thalamic organization has been established and the ventricular zone of the diencephalon has ceased neuron production. The source of the late-forming pulvinar cells was found in the nearby ganglionic eminence situated in the telencephalon. This transient developmental structure contains numerous proliferative cells throughout the last two trimesters, but had been thought by most previous investigators to give neurons exclusively for the basal ganglia, particularly the caudate nucleus. However, some young cells appear to stream from the ganglionic eminence, cross the ditelencephalic boundary beneath the sulcus terminalis, and enter the thalamus at the posterolateral surface of the pulvinar. The migratory cells form a densely packed cellular sheath designated as the corpus gangliothalamicum. The structure, approximately 200 $\mu$ wide and 2000 $\mu$ long was found consistently just under the external surface of the developing pulvinar of fetuses from 18 to 34 weeks of gestation. Golgi analysis revealed that many of these cells are migrating neurons, since the youngest 'bipolar forms are positioned nearest the ganglionic eminence and progressively more mature and complex ones lie deeper in the pulvinar. Thus the early proliferation-migration events in the wall of the third ventricle that characterize thalamic development in all mammals are supplemented in man by late and prolonged accretion of cells that arise in the ganglionic eminence of the telencephalon but take permanent residence in the neothalamus. The speculation was offered that the ganglionic eminence might supply simultaneously cells destined for the late-forming, functionally interconnected components of posterior neocortex and thalamus.

## References

Altman, J.: Autoradiographic and histological studies of postnatal neurogenesis. 11. A longitudinal investigation of the kinetics, migration and transformation of cells incorporating tritiated thymidine in infant rats, with special reference to postnatal neurogenesis in some brain regions. *J. Comp. Neur. 128:*431–473, 1966.

Angevine, J.B., Jr.: Time of neuron origin in the hippocampal region. An autoradiographic study in the mouse. *Exp. Neur., Supplement 2:*1–70, 1965.

Angevine, J.B., Jr.: Time of neuron origin in the diencephalon of the mouse. An autoradiographic study. *J. Comp. Neur. 139:*129–188, 1970a.

Angevine, J.B., Jr.: Critical cellular events in the shaping of neural centers. In F.O. Schmitt (Ed.), *The Neurosciences.* New York, The Rockefeller Univ. Press, pp. 60–72, 1970b.

Boulder Committee Embryonic vertebrate central nervous system: Revised terminology. *Anat. Rec. 166:*257–262, 1970.

Clark, W.E.L.: The structure and connections of the thalamus. *Brain, 55:*406–470, 1932.

Debakan, A.: Human thalamus. An anatomical developmental and pathological study. Development of the human thalamic nuclei. *J. Comp. Neur. 100:*63–97, 1954.

Dewulf, A.: *Anatomy of the Normal Human Thalamus.* Amsterdam: Elsevier, 196 pp, 1971.

Essick, C.R.: The development of the nuclei pontis and the nucleus arcuatus in man. *Am. J. Anat. 13:*25–54, 1912.

Flechsig, P.: *Anatomie des menschichen Gehirns and Rückenmarks auf myelogenetischer Grundlage.* Leipzig, George Thieme, 1920.

Frazer, J.E.: *A Manual of Embryology.* Second Edition. Chapter XI, The Nervous System. Baltimore, Williams & Wilkins, pp. 135–204, 1920.

Geschwind, N.: Disconnexion syndroms in animals and man. Part 1. *Brain:* 88:237–294, 1965.

Gilbert, M.: The early development of the human diencephalon. *J. Comp. Neur.* 62:81–115, 1934.

Graybiel, A.M.: Some ascending connections of the pulvinar and nucleus lateralis posterior of the thalamus in the cat. *Brain Res.* 44:99–125; 1972a.

Graybiel, A.M.: Some fiber pathways related to the posterior thalamic region in the cat. *Brain, Behavior and Evolution,* 6:363-393

Hamilton, W.J., Boyd, J.D., and Mossman, H.W.: *Human Embryology.* 3rd Ed. Baltimore, Williams & Wilkins, 1952.

Hassler, R.: Functional anatomy of the thalamus. In: *6th Latin-Amer. Congr. of Neurosurgery,* Montevideo, pp. 754–787, 1955.

Herrick, C.J.: The morphology of the forebrain in Amphibia and Reptilia. *J. Comp. Neur.* 20:413–547, 1910.

Hinds, J.W.: Autoradiographic study of histogenesis in the mouse olfactory bulb. 1. Time of origin of neurons and neuroglia. *J. Comp. Neur.* 134:287–304, 1968.

Hochstetter, F.: *Beitrage zur Entwicklungsgeschichte des menschlichen Gehirus.* Vienna and Lepsig, Franz Deuticke, 1919.

Kahle, W.: Zue Entwicklung des menschlichen Zwischenhirs. *Dtsch. Z. Nervenheilk.* 175:259–318, 1956.

Källén, B.: Embryological studies on the neuclei and their homogenization in the vertebrate forebrain. *Kungl. Fysiogrfisra Sallskapets Hondliuger,* N.F. 62:3–34, 1951.

Karten, J.H.: The organization of the avian telencephalon and some speculations on the phylogeny of the amniote telencephalon. *Ann. N.Y. Acad. Sci.* 167:164–179, 1969.

Marin–Padilla, M.: Early prenatal ontogenesis of the cerebral cortex (Neocortex) of the cat (Felis Domestica). A Golgi Study. 1. The primordial neocortical organization. *Z. Anat. Entwick.-Gesch.* 134:117–145, 1971.

McLardy, T.: Thalamic microneurons. *Nature,* 199:820–821, 1963.

Miale, I. and Sidman, R.L.: An autoradiographic analysis of histogenesis in the mouse cerebellum. *Exptl. Neur.* 4:277–296, 1961.

Miura, R.: Über die Differenzierung des Grundbestandteile in Zwischenhirn des Kaninchens. *Anat. Anz.* 77:1–65, 1933.

von Monakow, C.: Experimentelle und pathologisch-anatomische Untersuchungen über die Hanbenregion, den Sehhugel und die Regio subthalamica, nebst Beitragen zur Kenntniss früh erworbener Gross-und Kleinhirndefekte. *Arch. Psychiat. Nervenkr.* 27:1–128, 386–478, 1895.

Morest, D.K.: A study of neurogenesis in the forebrain of opposum pouch young. Z. *Anat. Etwickl.-Gesch. 130:*265–305, 1970.

Niimi, K., Harada, I., Kuska, Y., and Kishi, S.: The ontogenetic development of the diencephalon of the mouse. *Tokushima J. Exp. Med. 8:*203–238, 1962.

Patten, B.M.: *Human Embryology. 2nd Ed.* Toronto, Blakiston, 1953.

Poliakov, G.I.: Some results of research into the development of the neuronal structure of the cortical ends of the analyzers in man. *J. Comp. Neur. 117:*197–212, 1961.

Poliakov, G.I.: Development of the cerebral neocortex during first half of. intrauterine life. (In Russian) In S.A. Sarkisov (Ed.) *Development of the Child's Brain.* Leningrad, Medicina, pp. 22–52, 1965.

Ramon y Cajal, S.: *Studies on Vertebrate Neurogenesis.* (L. Guth, transl.). Springfield, Charles C Thomas, 1960.

Rakic, P.: Neuron-glia relationship during granule cell migration in developing cerebellar cortex. A Golgi and electronmicroscopic study in macacus rhesus. *J. Comp. Neur. 141:*283–312, 1971.

Rakic, P.: Mode of cell migration to the superficial layers of fetal monkey neocortex. *J. Comp. Neur. 145:*61–84, 1972.

Rakic, P.: Kinetics of the proliferation and the latency between final division and onset of differentiation of the cerebellar stellate and basket cells. *J. Comp. Neuro. 147:*523–546; 1973a.

Rakic, P. and Sidman, R.L.: Supravital DNA synthesis in the developing human and mouse brain. *J. Neuropath. Exptl. Neurol. 27:*246–272, 1969.

Rakic, P. and Sidman, R.L.: Telencephalic origin of pulvinar neurons in the fetal human brain. Z. *Anat. Entwickl.-Gesch. 129:*53–82, 1969.

Rose, J.E.: The ontogenetic development of the rabbit's diencephalon. *J. Comp. Neur. 77:*61–129, 1942.

Scheibel, E.M., Davies, T.L., and Scheibel, A.B.: An unusual axonless cell in the thalamus of the adult cat. *Exp. Neurol. 36:*512–518; 1972.

Schaper, A.: Die frühensten Differenzirungsvorgänge im Centralnerven system. *Arch. F. Entwichelungs-Mechanik. 5:*81–132, 1897.

Sidman, R.L.: Histogenesis of mouse retina studied with thymidine-$H^3$, In G.K. Smelser (Ed.) *The Structure of the Eye.* New York, Academic Press, pp. 487–506, 1961.

Sidman, R.L.: Cell proliferation, migration and interaction in the developing mammalian central nervous system. In F.O. Schmitt (Ed.) *The Neurosciences. Second Study Program.* New York, Rockefeller Univ. Press, pp. 100–107, 1970.

Smith, G.E.: Some problems relating to the evolution of the Brain. *Lancet, 1:*1–6; 147–153; 221–227, 1910.

30     *The Pulvinar-LP Complex*

Taber-Pierce, E.: Histogenesis of the nuclei griseum pontis, corporis pontobulbaris and reticularis tegmenti pontis (Bechterew) in the mouse. An autoradiographic study. *J. Comp. Neur.* 126:219–240, 1966.

Taber-Pierce, E.: Histogenesis of the dorsal and ventral cochlear nuclei in the mouse. An autoradiographic study. *J. Comp. Neur.* 131:27–38, 1967.

Windle, W.F.: Development of neural elements in human embryos of four to seven weeks gestation. *Exp. Neurol.* Supp. 5:44–83, 1970.

Yakovlev, P.I.: The development of the nuclei of the dorsal thalamus and of the cerebral cortex; morphogenetic and tectogenetic correlation. In S. Locke (Ed.). *Modern Neurology.* Papers in tribute to Professor Derek Denny-Brown. New York, Little, Brown & Co., 1967.

Yakovlev, P.I. and Lecours, A.R.: The myelogenetic cycles of regional maturation of the brain. In A. Minkowski (Ed.) *Regional Development of the Brain in Early Life.* Oxford and Edinburgh, Blackwell Scientific Publications, pp. 3–70, 1967.

## ACKNOWLEDGMENT

This research was supported in part by NIH grant 5–R01–NS09081 to the Department of Neuropathology, Harvard Medical School, and by grant PL–480–02–006 from the NIH (USA) to the Institute of Biological Research and Center for Multidisciplinary Postgraduate Studies, Belgrade University. I am grateful to Prof. Dr. V. Šulović, University Gynecological Hospital, Belgrade, Yugoslavia for providing fresh human specimens for supravital autoradiography, Golgi analysis and electronmicroscopy. I also thank Dr. P.I. Yakovlev, W.E. Fernald State School, Boston, Mass. for access to cases of serially sectioned human fetal brains.

## DISCUSSION

**Dr. Cooper:** I'm sure that anyone who has not read Dr. Rakic's work before could see why this elegant, meticulous study is so exciting. During our own recent work on the pulvinar, we wondered whether the pulvinar might not be better considered as a part of the basal ganglia. One of the reasons has been his remarkable piece of work but another very simple one is the close apposition of the body of the caudate to the pulvinar which in sagittal section makes them look almost like one structure. I wonder what you think about anatomical relationship between caudate and pulvinar and their relationship to cortex? It is conceivable that we are justified in thinking of them as one structure?

**Dr. Rakic:** No, I wouldn't say so. They are distinct anatomical entities. The point in common established from developmental analysis is that both structures are embryologically related to the ganglionic eminence. Both the basal ganglia and the pulvinar receive neurons from the same or closely related areas of the proliferative zone situated in the ventricular wall of the telencephalon. The anlage of the caudate nucleus is virtually embedded in the ganglionic eminence and this is perhaps the reason why in most textbooks the entire ganglionic eminence is marked as a prospective caudate nucleus. The evidence reviewed today indicates that the ganglionic eminence at one point in time "exports" cells to the posterior thalamus. It should be emphasized that early formed neurons of both pulvinar and LP appear to be of diencephalic origin. Therefore only some cells, and we don't know how many, have migrated to the pulvinar from the telencephalon. The fact that both the caudate nucleus and the pulvinar at one point in ontogeny receive cells from the same general source has unknown significance.

**Dr. Trachetenberg:** I have the impression, and I want to make sure that it's not incorrect, that a large number of the cells entering the pulvinar from the ganglionic eminence find their way towards the posteriormost portions of the pulvinar that part that extends into the transverse fissure. So could we conclude that the rostral parts of the medial pulvinar don't get the benefit of these cells?

**Dr. Rakic:** No, I think that would be a wrong interpretation. I have emphasized that most cells of telencephalic origin are going to the posterior part of the thalamus because we have seen transitional forms in this region. The analysis of the Golgi material was crucial for this interpretation. Cells in the corpus gangliothalamicum are bipolar as they migrate. Later on as they move from the posterior thalamic surface both deeper and more medially into the pulvinar, some cells become more complex in form. Their shape changes from bipolar to multipolar, and they become fixed in position. However, it is possible that some cells migrate much deeper and even pass more anteriorly into the posterior part of the nucleus medialis dorsalis. Unfortunately, Golgi material was available only in the posterior part of the pulvinar and we are not sure how far anteriorly some cells might migrate. We hope to gain such information by tracing cells of the ganglionic eminence tagged with thymidine-H[3] label in rhesus monkeys. Naturally, the analysis will work only if this species has the population of cells in question. Hitherto, the corpus gangliothalamicum has been observed only in humans. It has not been seen in rabbit, mouse, or opossum, and has not been sought so far in fetal monkeys.

**Dr. Frigyesi:** Do you think that neuron cells in the ganglionic eminence represent the primordium for the entire caudate nucleus or only for the head of the caudate nucleus? The distinction ought to be made because the head of the caudate nucleus has been shown to be a component of the sensory-motor organization, whereas the body and the tail of the caudate nucleus, have not been included in this organization. The second question: Is there any evidence that the ganglionic eminence represents at least in part, the primordium for other parts of the basal ganglia such as the globus pallidus, putamen, claustrum?

**Dr. Rakic:** The answer to the first question is affirmative. Probably the entire caudate receives cells from the ganglionic eminence. So also does the putamen and even the amygdala and parts of the septal nuclear complex.

**Dr. Frigyesi:** What about globus pallidus?

**Dr. Rakic:** The developmental history of the globus pallidus is very interesting. Its lateral portion probably receives a large number of cells from the ganglionic eminence. However, the cells of the medial portion of globus pallidus are apparently of diencephalic origin. From the studies of Richter (1965) and Kukuev (1961, 1965), it seems that the medial portion of the globus pallidus originates in the ventral thalamus in a longitudinal band continuous with the subthalamic nucleus and zona incerta, and subsequently becomes shifted rostrally and laterally into the base of the telencephalon.

**Dr. Gilman:** Gentlemen, I wanted to clarify three issues. One is, is the pulvinar composed only of cells from the ventricular wall, the ganglionic eminence and the corpus gangliothalamicum or are there additional contributions from the other embryonic structures? The second question which you already partially answered is: to what other structures does the ganglionic eminence contribute besides the caudate and the lateral portion of the globus pallidus? Are there other parts of diencephalon, for example, which receive cells from it? Thirdly, what is the source of the corpus gangliothalamicum? CGT in one of your slides I believe. Does it receive cells from the ganglionic eminence?

**Dr. Rakic:** That's right. The corpus gangliothalamicum as seen in any given fixed fetal specimen, contains cells migrating at that particular moment in time from the ganglionic eminence. The structure is constantly present for several months, but comprises a constantly changing cell population in transit from ganglionic eminence to thalamus. It contains very few proliferating cells.

**Dr. Gilman:** Well, I just wanted to clarify that issue, and to find out whether in fact the pulvinar really has two sources: one, the diencephalic ventricular wall; and the second, the telencephalic ganglionic eminence.

**Dr. Rakic:** Exactly, it does have two sources.

**Dr. Gilman:** On the other hand, a large part of the basal ganglia in turn comes from the ganglionic eminence, so does this structure represent the important primordial source for a large part of the telencephalon?

**Dr. Rakic:** That's right. I think you almost completely answered your own questions at the end. The only remaining question is whether the thalamus gets cells also from some third source. I don't believe so, for there seems to be no proliferative site from which to get them. Only these two germinal sources are available. Until recently we knew only of one, and this is the ventricular zone, or matrix zone, of the third ventricle. Now we can add the second one, the ganglionic eminence in the floor of the lateral ventricles. I think you stated it very well that the ganglionic eminence represents the main source of neurons for large telencephalic structures such as basal ganglia, including amygdala. However, it should be emphasized that in man the ganglionic eminence persists to the end of gestation and even beyond birth. It is possible that particularly towards the end of its existence, it becomes a source of glia. After all, glia also have to come from somewhere. We are usually concerned very much about formation of neuronal sets and forget that there is an equal or even larger number of "supportive" cells in the brain.

**Dr. Poirier:** I would like to add some comments that may help in understanding this relationship. As you first mentioned, the ganglionic eminence, a phylogenetically older structure, gives rise to the caudate nucleus and contributes to the septal nuclei, nucleus accumbens septi, etc. I am thinking of new approaches based on histochemistry that may prove useful in elucidating the topographical arrangement of different nervous elements within such structures. As a matter of fact, the structures you have mentioned, such as the septal nucleus and nucleus accumbens septi are particularly rich in cholinesterase and in this respect they have much in common with the caudate nucleus, the putamen and the external pallidum and, also, a peculiar zone of the amygdala. There is also a series of nuclei located in the caudal part of the diencephalon which display an intense cholinesterasic activity as shown by Olivier in our laboratory. This series of nuclei including nuclei limitans, suprageniculatus, peripeduncularis, etc, prolong caudally the reticular nucleus of the thalamus and also extend towards the intralaminar nucleus as may be disclosed on horizontal and sagittal sections of the brain of the cat and monkey. Therefore, I wonder whether these structures could not be made up of cells that have migrated from the ganglionic eminence, as all these structures show an intense and uniform cholinesterasic activity. I think this peculiar topographical distribution of the enzyme may prove useful to determine a possible relationship between these structures.

**Dr. Rakic:** You're quite right. There is a study by Krnjević and Silver (1966) in which they indeed showed cells with cholinesterase activity emerging from the ganglionic eminence and contributing also, interestingly enough, to the posterior part of the thalamus as well as to the portions of basal ganglia that you mentioned and to the parietal portion of the neocortex.

**Dr. Cooper:** Thank you Dr. Rakic. It is evident that Dr. Rakic has opened our meeting with a very stimulating and rich presentation. Dr. Siqueira has for several years been studying the anatomic relationships of the pulvinar and his presentation follows well on this developmental study.

## References

Krnjević, K. & Silver, A.: Acetylcholinesterase in the developing forebrain. *J. Anat.* (London), *100*:63–89, 1966.

Kukuev, L.A.: On the development of the motor analysor in man's ontogenesis. (in Russian. In S.A. Sarkisov (Ed.) *Structure and Function of the Analysors During Human Ontogenesis.* Moscow, Medgiz, pp. 257–263, 1961.

Kukuev, L.A.: Precentral area. Striopallidum, red nucleus, substantia nigra, corpus Luysi. (In Russian). In S.A. Sarkisov (Ed.) *Development of Child's Brain.* Leningrad, Medicina, pp. 160–173, 1965.

Richter, E.: Die Entwicklung des Globus pallidus und des Corpus Subthalamicus. *Monographien aus dem Gesamtgebiete der Neurologie und Psychiatrie, 108*:1–131, 1965.

---

# CHAPTER 2

# ANATOMIC CONNECTIONS OF THE PULVINAR

E.B. Siqueira, M.D., L. Franks, M.D.

## I. INTRODUCTION

THE NUCLEUS PULVINARIS is one of the largest nuclei of the dorsal thalamus in the primate. It has a complex anatomic structure. As a working hypothesis, it is presumed that its functions are as important as its size leads one to believe. D. Albe-Fessard and her associates (D. Albe-Fessard, et. al., 1963; J. Taren, et. al., 1968) have found that the pulvinar displays a characteristic spontaneous electrical activity, thus stressing the individuality of this nucleus. Its electrical stimulation has been associated with disturbances of speech in humans (G.A. Ojemann, et. al., 1968a; 1968b). This fact indicates that this nucleus is related to the so-called "higher functions" of the human brain. New interest has centered in this nucleus since it was demonstrated that its destruction is an effective means of abolishing abnormal movements (I.S. Cooper, et. al., 1971). The precise role, or roles, of the nucleus, however, is not clear at the present time.

As early as 1894, E. Brissaud, as quoted by J. Déjerine (1901), was concerned with the connections of the pulvinar and described fibers projecting from the temporal cortex into

¹ This research was supported in part by Grant #NB–08968 from the National Institute of Neurological Diseases and Stroke, the Training Grant #NB–5408 from the National Institute of Health, and the Program Project Grant #NS–09377 from the National Institute of Health.

the pulvinar. These connections have since been confirmed by several investigators (refer to references mentioned in E. Siqueira, 1965).

Phylogenetically the pulvinar is first recognized in the opossum (Didelphis virginiana), though it has been questioned whether it is truly separated from the pretectal nucleus (C. Tsai, 1925). In the armadillo the pulvinar is more defined (J. W. Papez, 1932). Many well circumscribed subnuclei are found in the rat (E. Gurdjian, 1927). This evolutive process appears to progress sequentially from rabbit, to cat and to dog in which species the divisions, as identified in the primates, become apparent (G.W. Papez, 1932).

The present knowledge of the pulvinar connections with other parts of the brain is based largely on patterns of degeneration following cerebral cortical lesions. Few studies have been based on lesions placed in the pulvinar itself. R. Crouch (1940) placed single lesions in the pulvinars of each of three monkeys and studied the degenerating fibers arising from these lesions. In two animals the lesions involved the medial portion of the pulvinar. Degenerating fibers arising from these lesions were found to comprise two distinct groups. One group consisted of medially directed fibers. They entered the midbrain. The second group consisted of laterally directed fibers. They entered the temporal lobe. In the third animal the lesions involved the lateral portion of the pulvinar. From this lesion fibers were distributed as the fibers originating from the medially placed lesion. K. Chow (1954) made bilateral stereotactic lesions in the pulvinars of several monkeys. K. Chow, however, did not investigate the degenerating fibers, which may have arisen from the lesion. Recently R.T. Thompson and R. Myers (1971) made bilateral lesions in the pulvinar of four monkeys. They confined their investigation, however, to the study of behavioral changes.

In the present study the patterns of degeneration resulting from well controlled lesions, surgically placed in the pulvinars of monkeys, have been examined in an attempt to better establish the connections of the pulvinar with the cerebral cortex and subcortical nuclei.

## II. METHODS OF STUDY

Tables I and II give the histological techniques as well as the lesions performed in the animals comprising the subject of this presentation. All animals were adult Rhesus monkeys weighing six to ten pounds.

TABLE I
STAINING METHODS USED

| | |
|---|---|
| *Group I* | |
| Control animals | — 3 animals |
| Stains used: Nissl and Woelcke | |
| *Group II* | |
| Animals used for calibration of stereotaxic apparatus | — 3 animals |
| Stain used: Nissl (frozen section) | |
| *Group III* | |
| Animals sacrificed 10–30 days following placement of the lesions | — 50 animals |
| Stains used: Marchi—30 animals | |
| Nauta—20 animals | |
| *Group IV* | |
| Animals sacrificed from several months to few years following placement of the lesions | — 7 animals |
| Stains used: Nissl and Woelcke | |
| *Group V* | |
| Animals used for evaluation of pulvinar lesions created by the "open" method | — 10 animals |
| Stain used: Nissl (frozen section) | |
| TOTAL—73 | |

NOTE: Actual total of animals: 71. Two animals are counted twice as they had occipital lesions on one side and parietal lesions on opposite side.

TABLE II
LESIONS

| | |
|---|---|
| Control animals | 3 animals |
| Calibration of sterotaxic apparatus | 3 animals |
| Evaluation of "open" pulvinar lesions | 10 animals |
| Hemispherectomies | 4 animals |
| Hemidecortication | 1 animal |
| Isolated lesions | |
| Complete temporal lobectomy | 11 animals |
| Temporal decortication (partial or complete) | 4 animals |
| Deep temporal lesions | 2 animals |
| Lesions in the occipital lobe | |
| Lobectomies | 9 animals |
| Occipital decortication (parietal) | 5 animals |
| Lesions in the parietal lobe | 6 animals |
| Lesions in the frontal lobe (lobectomies) | 2 animals |
| Section of the optic nerve | 4 animals |
| Lesions in the pulvinar (stereotaxic placement) | 9 animals |
| TOTAL—73 | |

NOTE: Actual total of animals: 71. Two animals are counted twice as they had occipital lesions on one side and parietal lesions on opposite side.

### III RESULTS

## I. The pulvinar and its subdivisions

Three divisions of the pulvinar are distinguished (Walker, 1938): the nucleus pulvinaris medialis, the nucleus pulvinaris lateralis and the nucleus pulvinaris inferior (fig. 1).

## II. Changes in the pulvinar following hemidecortications and hemispherectomies

Four hemispherectomized animals were studied. These animals were sacrificed following a survival time of respectively 4, 9, and 12 months, and 5 years. In all these animals there was complete degeneration of the neuronal elements in the pulvinar homolateral to the hemispherectomy.

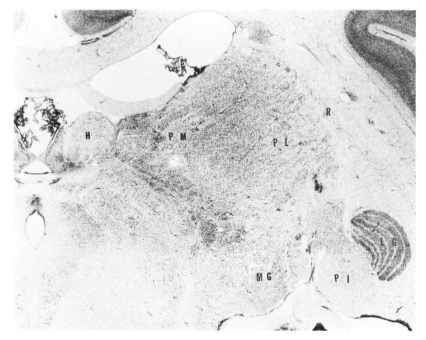

Figure 2–1. Coronal section through the anterior portion of the pulvinar. PM: Pulvinaris medialis; PL: pulvinaris lateralis; PI: pulvinaris inferior; LG: lateral geniculate; MG: medial geniculate; R: reticularis; H: habenula. (Nissl stain).

One animal underwent a hemidecortication. He was sacrificed 3 years later. In this animal there was also a complete disappearance of all the neurons of the pulvinar.

### III. Changes in the pulvinar following isolated cortical lesions

1. *Changes in the pulvinar following temporal lobectomy* (Siqueira, 1965)

These changes are characterized by intense gliosis and neuronal loss in the animals which were left to survive for a prolonged period of time. The animals which were sacrificed within two to four weeks following the temporal lobectomy showed intense degeneration in Marchi and Nauta preparations. The degeneration was very intense and confined mostly to the postero-medial part of the pulvinar.

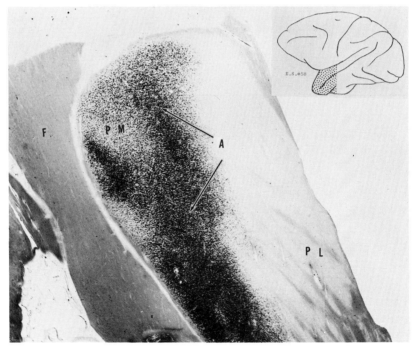

Figure 2–2. Coronal section through the pulvinar showing degeneration (arrows A) following a lesion limited to area 38. The extent of this resection is shown in the inset. PM: pulvinaris medialis; PL: pulvinaris lateralis; F: fornix. (Marchi method).

2. *Changes in the pulvinar following temporal decortication (partial or complete)* (Siqueira, 1965)

In these animals the resection was limited to the neocortex of the temporal lobe. In every instance the pulvinar revealed degeneration which was more pronounced in or confined to the medial posterior portion of the nucleus. This projection was heaviest from area 38 (figs. 2,3,4 and 5).

3. *Changes in the pulvinar following lesion in the occipital lobe*

Marchi preparations of animals which had undergone extensive lobectomies showed large degenerating fibers traversing the pulvinar on their way to the tectal region. Besides these cortico-tectal fibers there was also degeneration involving

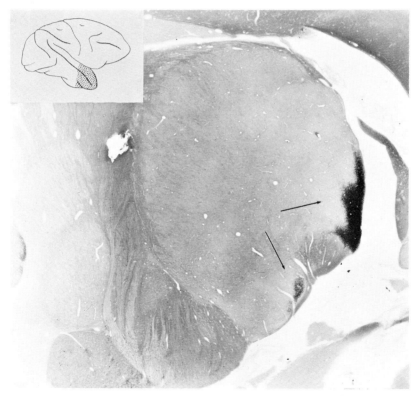

Figure 2–3. Parasagittal section through the pulvinar to demonstrate degeneration (arrows) following partial resection of the temporal cortex. The extent of this resection is shown in the inset. (Marchi method).

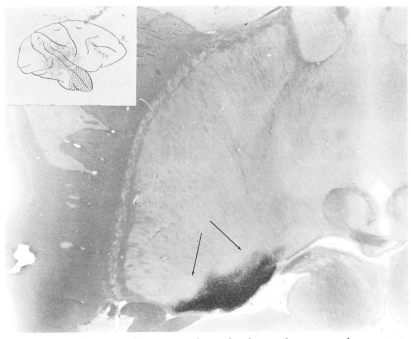

Figure 2–4. Horizontal section through the pulvinar to demonstrate degeneration (arrows) following partial resection of the temporal cortex. The extent of this resection is shown in the inset. (Marchi method).

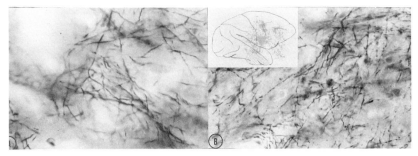

Figure 2–5. Nauta preparations (high power magnification) of the pulvinar. This animal underwent a resection of the anterior portion of the right temporal lobe. The extent of this resection is shown in the inset. (A) Left pulvinar to be compared with the right pulvinar (B) which demonstrates segmentation of the axons.

the pulvinar itself, thus demonstrating the termination of other fibers in this nucleus. This degeneration which was more pronounced anteriorly, was confined to the most lateral and inferior portions of the pulvinar (fig. 6). Degeneration in the pulvinar, however, was not present in all animals. Analysis of the lesions indicated that the monkeys in which degeneration in the pulvinar had been encountered presented involvement of the anterior portion of the occipital cortex with encroachment upon the parietal or temporal lobes or upon both of these lobes. There had been also partial destruction or undermining of the posteriormost portion of the temporal lobe. In one of the animals there was also slight destruction of the most dorsal and posterior portion of the parietal cortex. The animals in which the cortex of the lunate sulcus (anterior occipital cortex) was spared did not present any degeneration of the pulvinar. Nauta preparations confirmed the findings described above in the Marchi impregnations.

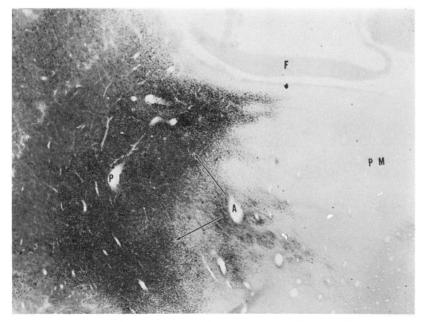

Figure 2–6. Coronal section through the pulvinar showing degeneration (arrows A) following extensive occipital lobectomy. PM: pulvinaris medialis; PL: pulvinaris lateralis; F: fornix. (Marchi method).

After the results described above became available, it was decided to demonstrate that even the anteriormost portion of area 17 does not project to the pulvinar: this hypothesis was confirmed in 3 animals (each one with 2 lesions) which were studied with the Nauta technique. Interesting enough, in all these animals the cortico-tectal fibers could be clearly seen crossing the pulvinar on their way to the tectal area where they terminated around cellular groups. These fibers, however, did not give any terminations in the pulvinar itself.

Evaluating the combined results of these animals, it can be concluded that at least the convexity of area 17 does not project to the pulvinar. This applies even to the most anterior portion of this area. The sulcal cortex of the lunate sulcus (areas 18 and 19) does project to the pulvinar however. The projection is very slight and only massive lesions of area 18 and 19 produce easily detectable degeneration in the pulvinar. In the only case in which this degeneration was extensive the most dorsal and posterior part of the parietal cortex was also involved. In this animal the posteriormost portion of the temporal lobe was also decorticated. In every case in which degeneration was present in the pulvinar it was confined to the most anterior and inferior portion of the pulvinaris lateralis. In two additional animals in which small lesions were confined to the sulcal cortex of the lunate sulcus no degeneration was present in the pulvinar. Apparently the connections between area 18 and 19 with the pulvinar are not very dense. They can be demonstrated by the Nauta technique only when the lesions have been extensive.

4. *Changes in the pulvinar following lesions in the parietal lobe*

In these animals there was no evidence of degeneration in the pulvinar despite the fact that some of the lesions were very extensive. The specimens obtained were impregnated either with the Marchi or with the Nauta techniques. It was interesting to observe the parieto-tectal fibers coursing through the pulvinar without releasing any termination in this nucleus.

5. *There was no evidence of degeneration in the pulvinar even after very extensive frontal lobectomies.*

## IV. Changes in the pulvinar following lesions in the optic nerves

The animals which were studied following section of the optic nerve failed to reveal any degeneration in the pulvinar.

## V. Degeneration observed following lesions placed in pulvinar

### 1. *Unilateral lesions* (Siqueira, 1968)

These lesions were placed stereotactically. In each animal just one lesion was made. The specimens obtained were impregnated either by the Marchi or by the Nauta technique. The lesions were placed in the nucleus pulvinaris medialis (fig. 7) or in the nucleus pulvinaris lateralis. No lesions were placed in the nucleus pulvinaris inferior. The most striking finding encountered in studying the degeneration resulting from these lesions was the sparseness of degenerating fibers arising from the lesion. This is in sharp contrast to the heavy degeneration localized to these same areas resulting from lesions involving the temporal lobe. Despite the sparseness and the poor impregnation of the fine degenerating pulvino-temporal fibers, they could be followed on their way to the temporal lobe. They reached the internal capsule either crossing through the dorsal or through the midportion of the pulvinar. After reaching the internal capsule they coursed ventrally to enter the white matter of the temporal lobe. These fibers entered gradually the cortex of the temporal lobe.

### 2. *Large lesions placed bilaterally in the pulvinar.*

In our present study of behavioral changes consequent to bilateral pulvinarectomy, we have been disappointed in our attempt to obtain complete and yet well circumscribed lesions within this pear-shaped nucleus by the closed method of stereotactic electrocoagulation. Solitary large lesions have resulted in variable degrees of damage to adjacent brain stem tissue. Multiple small electrolytic lesions require multiple passes of the electrode through neocortex and corpus callosum and seldom destroy the entire pulvinar. A series of bilateral pulvinarectomies has been performed by an open aspiration technique.

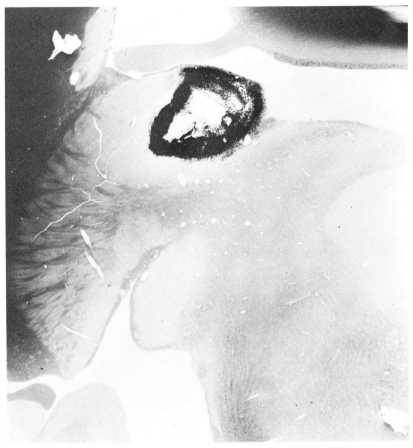

Figure 2–7. Coronal section through pulvinar to demonstrate lesion stereotactically produced. (Marchi method).

*Technique* (fig. 8) The operation is performed under general anesthesia. Mannitol (20% "Osmitrol"), two grams per kilogram, is administered by slow intravenous bolus injection prior to placing the animal in a standard laboratory operating frame. The operation is carried out under sterile conditions. A transverse biparietal scalp incision is made from tragus to tragus. The scalp flaps are retracted to expose almost the entire calvarium. To achieve adequate mobilization of the hemispheres without contusing the cortex, large parieto-occipital bone flaps hinged to the temporal muscles are

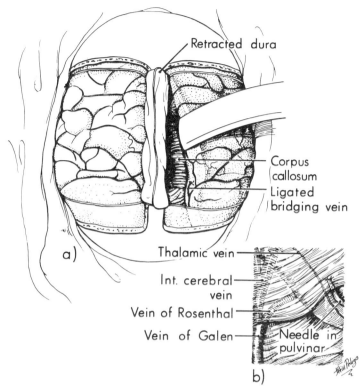

Figure 2–8. a) Diagramatic view of operative exposure. b) Introducing bent needle (arrow) into pulvinar lateral to the surface thalamic vein.

turned. A bony ridge is left overlying the superior sagittal sinus for support of the bone flaps on closure. Bilateral dural flaps are made and reflected medially. The approach consists of retracting the hemispheres laterally and away from the falx cerebri, thus exposing the posterior thalamus in the midline. A constant cortical bridging vein overlying the parietal lobe is coagulated and sectioned. Occasionally a second bridging vein from the occipital pole is also cut. We have never found it necessary to section or coagulate blood vessels other than these two for adequate mobilization of the hemispheres. The parietal lobe is then patiently and gently retracted laterally exposing the splenium of the corpus callosum. The vein of Galen is identified beneath this structure. The operating

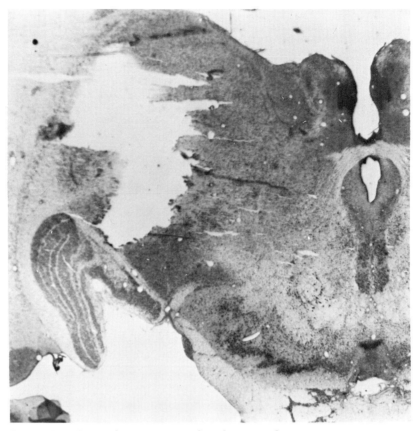

Figure 2–9. Coronal section trrough pulvinar to demonstrate anterior portion of lesion produced by the "open approach."

microscope is used for the remainder of the procedure. Using sharp dissection arachnoid trabeculae adhering to the retrosplenial neocortex, the posterior hippocampus, the great vein of Galen, converging cerebellar veins, and the midbrain tectum are freed. Adequate lysis of these trabeculae is necessary for retraction of the retrosplenial cortex overlying the dorsal thalamus. The bulge of the pulvinar is identified superolateral to the tectum. A surface thalamic vein is constantly present, and it is a useful reference structure; it indicates that the pulvinar has been adequately exposed. With a sharpe knife the pia mater is incised lateral to the above noted thalamic vein. Incising medial to this vessel increases the danger of damaging the underlying lateral geniculate body. A three inch, 16 gauge, blunt needle attached to very low suction is then inserted through the pial opening. Ablation of the antero-medial portion of the nucleus has been facilitated by bending the needle. Various angled drawn glass tubing also worked well. The needle is inserted 5 mm anteriorly. Care is taken on directing the aspirator inferiorly lest the lateral geniculate body be damaged. Minimal oozing of blood usually subsides spontaneously. The surgical wound is closed in anatomical layers. Penicillin is given prophylactically for three days. No infection has occurred in our series. The illustrations presented represent coronal sections through the pulvinar (figs. 9 and 10). The contour of the lesion varies with that of the target. Thus the integrity of the lateral geniculate body, internal capsule, and midbrain tegmentum has been preserved despite the size of the lesion.

Preliminary behavioral testing of the animals which have undergone bilateral extensive destruction of the pulvinar has shown impairment of function characterized by a slowness in learning. It has also been difficult to train these animals for visual testing.

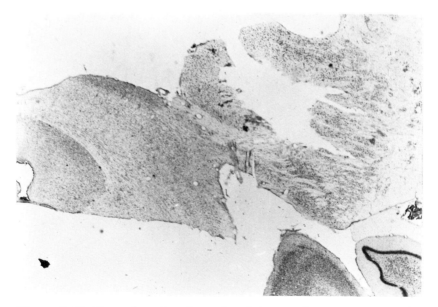

Figure 2–10. Coronal section through pulvinar to demonstrate posterior portion of lesion produced by the "open approach."

## SUMMARY

1.  The connections of the nucleus pulvinaris of the dorsal thalamus are confined mainly to the cortex as there is complete neuronal loss and gliosis following ipsilateral hemispherectomy or hemidecortication. Collaterals to other thalamic nuclei or to the basal ganglia and brain stem cannot be excluded however. The problem of collaterals can be investigated by electrophysiological means. Anatomical approaches are not proper for such a study.

2.  There are dense connections between the temporal cortex and the pulvinar. These connections are denser with the more anterior parts of the temporal cortex. Area 38 seems to have the densest projections. Reciprocal connections (pulvino-temporal fibers) are present as one would expect. but they are very light. Apparently the pulvino-temporal fibers arising from the postero-medial tip of the pulvinar project mostly, if not exclusively, to the temporal pole.

3.  The temporal cortex is related mainly to the postero-medial part of the nucleus pulvinaris, that is: postero-medial part of the pulvinaris medialis and pulvinaris inferior.

4.  The occipital cortex is related mainly to the antero-lateral part of the nucleus pulvinaris: anterior part of the pulvinaris lateralis and pulvinaris inferior.

5.  Projections to the pulvinar from the anterior portion of the parietal lobe are either non-existent or very scarce.

6.  The pulvinar is not connected either directly nor mainly with any of the primary sensory systems. Its main or direct connections are with associative areas of the cortex.

7.  Considering the facts enumerated above, an insight regarding the functions of the pulvinar can be outlined: this nucleus must have associative functions. It is very possible that these associative functions are mostly related to the visual system.

8.  Following bilateral extensive pulvinarectomies, Rhesus monkeys have a slowness in learning. It has also been difficult to train animals for visual testing.

## References

Albe-Fessard, E., Arfel, G., Guiot, G.: Activites electriques caracteristiques de quelques structures cerebrales chez l'homme. *Annales de Chirurgie,* *17:*1185–1214,.1963.

Brissaud, E.: Du faisceaus dit "bandelette sous-optique" dans le racine posterieure du thalamus. *Nouvelle Iconographie de la Salpetriere,* 99–101, 1894.

Chow, K. L.: Lack of behavioral effects following destruction of some thalamic association nuclei in monkey. *Arch. Neurol. Psychiat.,* *71:*762–771, 1954.

Cooper, I.S.: Personal Communication (1971) at the meeting of the Fulton Society.

Crouch, R.L.: The efferent fibers of the thalamus of *Macacus rhesus. J. Comp. Neurol., 72:*177–186, 1940.

Dejerine, J.: Anatomie des centre nerveus. *J. Reuff, Paris,* 2 vols., 1901.

Gurdjian, E.S.: The diencephalon of the albino rat. Studies on the brain of the rat No. 2. *J. Comp. Neurol., 43:*1–114, 1927.

Ojemann, G.A. and Fedio, P.: Effect on stimulation of the human thalamus and parietal and temporal white matter on short-term memory. *J. Neurosurg. 29:*51–59, 1968.

Ojemann, G.A., Fedio, P. and Van Buren, J.M.: Anomia from pulvinar and subcortical parietal stimulation. *Brain. 91:*99–116, 1968.

Papez, J.W.: The thalamic nuclei of the nine-banded armadillo (*Tatusia novemcinta*). *J. Comp. Neurol., 56:*49–103, 1932.

Siqueira, E.B.: The temporo-pulvinar connections in the Rhesus monkey. *Arch. Neurol., 13:*321–330, 1965.

Siqueira, E.B.: The cortical connections of the nucleus pulvinaris of the dorsal thalamus in the Rhesus monkey. *J. fur Hirnforschung,* *10:*478–498, 1968.

Taren, J., Guiot, G., Derome, P. and Trigo, J.C.: Hazards of sterotaxic thalamectomy. Added safety factor in corroborating X-ray target localization with neurophysiological methods. *J. Neurosurg., 29:*173–182, 1968.

Thompson, R. and Myers, R.E.: Brainstem mechanisms underlying visually guided responses in the Rhesus monkey. *J. Comp. and Physiol. Psych.* *74:* No. 3. 479–512, 1971.

Tsai, C.: The optic tracts and centers of the opposum, *Didelphis Virginiana. J. Comp. Neurol., 39:*173–216, 1925.

Walker, A.E.: *The Primate Thalamus.* Chicago, The University of Chicago Press, 1938.

INVITED DISCUSSION

## Some Electrohodological Considerations of the LP-Pulvinar Complex

### T.L. FRIGYESI, M.D.

The dorsolateral thalamus (DLT) represents the last frontier of the terra incognita within this large nuclear mass (Walker, 1966). The pulvinar and the nuclei lateralis dorsalis and posterior constitute the lateral nuclear group of the dorsal thalamus (Mettler, 1948). Morphological studies have revealed that DLT is reciprocally linked to extensive areas of the neocortex (Clüver, Campos-Ortega, 1969; Siqueira, 1965; Simma, 1957). Electrophysiological studies have suggested that reciprocal connections operate between DLT and the amygdala (Palestini, Borlone, Tejos, 1968), lateral geniculate body and superior colliculus (Armengol, Palestini, 1968) and that the optic tract is synaptically linked to DLT cells (Armengol, Palestini, 1968; Godfrained, Meulders, Veraart, 1969). Other aspects of structure-function characteristics of DLT are not known at present. Yet, the enormous phylogenetic development of DLT between rodents and man indicates that DLT is involved in higher integration of nervous activities (Simma, 1957). Recent studies have indicated that one of these integrative activities is exerted over the sensorimotor organization (Cooper, In Press). This is particularly perplexing because the sensorimotor cortex appears to be the only neocortical region which does not have connections with DLT (Siqueira, 1965). Furthermore, anatomical studies have failed to detect any connections between DLT and other identified components of the sensorimotor organization.

Data in the present report on intracellular recordings from DLT neurons show that several subcortical organizations, which regulate transmission in the thalamic relays of the cerebello-cortico-corticospinal projection system (Frigyesi, Purpura, 1964), are also synaptically linked to neurons in DLT.

The experiments were performed on locally anesthetised, succinylcholine paralyzed, encéphale isolé cats. The data pre-

characteristics observed in 9 out of the 19 DLT neurons during low-frequency EP stimulation. In these cells, EP stimulation polysynaptically elicited brief (10–20 msec) excitatory post-synaptic potentials (EPSPs) and succeeding prolonged (up to 100 msec) inhibitory postsynaptic potentials (IPSPs). These EP evoked alternating, rhythmic activities were essentially similar to those observed in VA-VL and CM-Pf neurons under similar conditions (Feldman, Purpura, 1970; Frigyesi, Machek, 1970). However, unlike in ventrolateral and medial thalamic neurons (Frigyesi, Rabin, 1971), evidence of EP evoked monosynaptic excitation of DLT neurons was not obtained.

The nine DLT neurons responsive to EP stimulation also generated polysynaptic EPSP-IPSP sequences to low-frequency MT stimulation (Fig. 13C). DLT neurons which were engaged by converging EP and MT synaptic pathways failed to generate synaptically evoked responses during low-frequency stimulation of the Cd (Fig. 13D).

Five out of the 19 DLT neurons which were unresponsive to EP and MT stimulation generated polysynaptic EPSP-IPSP sequences during low-frequency stimulation of Cd (figs. 14 and 15D). The first stimulus of a repetitive, low-frequency train to Cd elicited prominent IPSPs in these neurons with (fig. 15D) or without (fig. 14A) a detectable prior EPSP. This effect contrasts starkly with those observed in VL neurons under similar conditions (Frigyesi, Machek, 1971): in VL cells gradual buildup of synaptic potentials was observed during 8/sec stimulation of Cd (fig. 15A and B). Cd evoked IPSPs attenuated gradually (over a period of several hundred msec), as shown in fig. 14C, after cessation of Cd stimulation. Such slowly declining hyperpolarizations were unaffected by 8/sec MT stimulation which effectively evoked prominent recruiting responses in the motor cortex (fig. 14C). Cd evoked EPSPs in some DLT neurons elicited by the second and subsequent stimuli of an 8/sec train to Cd arose from a level of sustained hyperpolarization (fig. 14B) and therefore failed to reach the firing level of the neuron. In other DLT neurons, individual stimuli within an 8/sec train to Cd occasionally failed to evoke

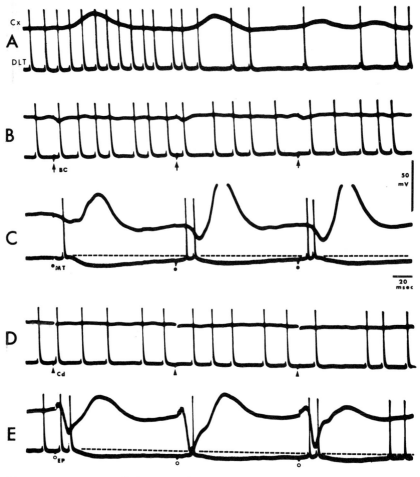

Figure 2–13. Intracellular recordings from a DLT neuron (lower traces). In this and subsequent figures, upper traces are surface recordings from the motor cortex (Cx). On the surface recordings, negativity is signaled by an upward deflection. Voltage calibrations relate to the intracellular traces. A, background activity. B, 8/sec stimulation of BC (at upward arrows) is ineffective in eliciting synaptic potentials in this neuron. C, 8/sec stimulation of MT elicits EPSP-IPSP sequences in this neuron coincident with prominent recruiting responses in the motor cortex. D, neuron is unresponsive to 8/sec stimulation of Cd (at arrow heads). E, 8/sec stimulation of EP elicits EPSP-IPSP sequences in this neuron. Note the absence of monosynaptic excitation of this neuron following the EP stimuli. The dashed horizontal lines are drawn through the assumed firing level of the neuron. (Modified from Frigyesi and Rabin, 1971).

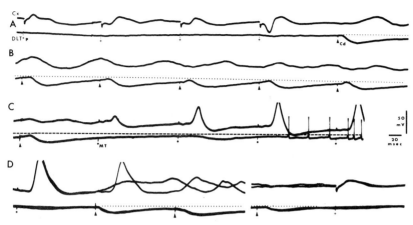

Figure 2–14. Sustained hyperpolarization elicited by Cd stimulation in a DLT neuron. A-C, continuous recordings. D, superimposed recordings. A, neuron is unresponsive to 8/sec stimulation of putamen (at crosses). Single shock to Cd elicits 10 msec latency prolonged IPSP. B, 8/sec Cd stimulation elicits EPSP-IPSP sequences. Dotted horizontal lines are drawn through the baseline membrane potential to emphasize that IPSP summation prevents evoked EPSPs from reaching the firing level. C, dashed horizontal line is drawn through the assumed firing level to show that the inhibitory aftereffects of Cd stimulation last 400 msec. Coincident 8/sec MT stimuli effectively generate recruiting responses in the motor cortex but fail to induce synaptic potentials in this neuron. D, left side, MT triggered spindle activities are seen in the motor cortex. Coincident Cd stimuli elicit synaptic potentials similar to those in A and B. Right side, after 600 msec, last stimulus of the 8/sec train to Cd elicits a prominent IP SP. Following abrupt switch to stimulation of putamen, synaptically evoked potentials are not demonstrable. (From: Frigyesi and Rabin, 1971).

detectable responses, yet the first Cd stimulus induced a sustained membrane polarization which was reinforced by some of the later evoked IPSPs; this resulted in suppression of spike generation during the entire period of 8/sec Cd stimulation (fig. 15D and E).

Coincident with spindle bursts in the motor cortex triggered by Cd stimulation, DLT neurons exhibited sequential alterations of the membrane potential similar to those observed in VL neurons (cf. Fig. 15C and E). Coincident with spindle bursts in the motor cortex triggered by MT stimulation, Cd effects in DLT neurons were similar to those observed under

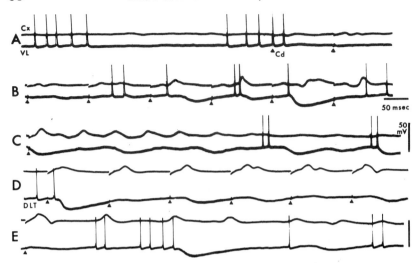

Figure 2–15. Comparison of Cd evoked activities in a DLT neuron (D and E) and in a VL neuron (A-C). A-C, and D-E, continuous recordings, respectively. A, background activity and initiation of 8/sec stimulation of Cd. B, repetitive Cd stimuli elicit typical incrementing "double-negativities" in the motor cortex and late developing EPSP-IPSP sequences in the VL neuron. C, cessation of 8/sec stimulation of Cd is followed by prominent and prolonged aftereffects at both recording sites. D, prominent EPSP-IPSP sequence in the DLT neuron is demonstrable following the first stimulus of an 8/sec train to Cd. E, "caudate spindle" in the motor cortical recording and triggered rhythmic activities in the DLT neuron are demonstrable following the cessation of Cd stimulation. (From: Frigyesi and Machek, 1971).

other conditions (cf. Fig. 14D and A). This lack of interaction between aftereffects of MT stimulation and Cd evoked synaptic potentials in DLT neurons contrasts sharply with observations in VL neurons: in VL, Cd and MT synaptic pathways interact (Frigyesi, Purpura, 1963).

The major finding in this report is the demonstration that synaptic pathways arising in Cd, EP and MT engage neurons in DLT. Electrical stimulation of these synaptic pathways elicit polysynaptic responses in DLT neurons similar to those observed in VA-VL and CM-Pf neurons under these conditions (Feldman, Purpura, 1970; Frigyesi, Machek, 1970; Frigyesi, Machek, 1971; Frigyesi, Purpura, 1963; Frigyesi, Purpura, 1964; Frigyesi, Rabin, 1971; Purpura, Cohen, 1962;

Purpura, Scarff, McMurtry, 1965). The major synaptic events in DLT neurons during low-frequency stimulation of Cd, EP and MT are alternating EPSPs and IPSPs. The duration of these evoked IPSPs (Feldman, Purpura, 1970) is three to four times longer than the duration of the evoked EPSPs. This results in prolonged suppression of spontaneous and evoked activities in DLT neurons and in interspersed brief periods during which evoked activities may be relayed through these neurons. Thus, low-frequency Cd, EP and MT stimulation induces synchronization of spontaneous and evoked activities in DLT neurons in much the same way as they do in ventrolateral and medial thalamic neurons (Frigyesi, Machek, 1970; Frigyesi, Machek, 1971; Frigyesi, Purpura, 1964; Frigyesi, Rabin, 1971; Purpura, Cohen, 1962; Purpura, Scarff, McMurtry, 1965). In certain instances, despite the alternation of evoked EPSPs and IPSPs, the evoked EPSPs were ineffective in triggering spike discharges because of the sustained hyperpolarization initiated by the first stimulus, most commonly Cd, in a repetitive low-frequency train. This resulted in suppression of spike generation during the entire period of stimulation, most frequently Cd. Similar prolonged Cd inhibition was observed in intracellular studies of EP neurons (Frigyesi, Machek, 1971).

A notable feature of DLT neurons, which emerged in this study, was a lack of convergence between EP and Cd projections. These findings corroborate a previous proposition which suggested that the major discharge route of Cd evoked excitatory activities to the dorsal thalamus is not via ansa lenticularis but through mesencephalic (SN) relays (Frigyesi, Machek, 1971).

These results indicate that the synaptic pathways which engage relay cells in the ventrolateral and medial thalamus and which regulate transmission through these neuronal elements also engage DLT neurons and generate essentially similar synaptic potentials in these cells. However, it is emphasized that those projections which generated monosynaptic excitation in VA-VL and CM-Pf neurons (BC, EP, and SN) (Frigyesi, Machek, 1970; Frigyesi, Machek, 1971;

Frigyesi, Rabin, 1971) failed to do so in DLT neurons. This indicates that DLT neurons are linked to various components of the sensorimotor organization through more complex multineuronal systems than neurons in the ventrolateral and medial thalamus.

These data which show medial thalamic synaptic pathways engaging DLT neurons will be corroborated by Richardson's data presented later in this symposium. He will demonstrate that peripheral evoked potentials in pulvinar may be abolished by lesions to medial thalamic nuclei. Thus medial thalamic nuclei may have a dual role regarding DLT functions: 1. its constituent neurons may relay information from the periphery (and from other sources?) to DLT; and 2. generate effects which regulate transmission through DLT neurons.

Cooper has recently reported that lesions to the LP-pulvinar complex alleviated certain abnormal sensorimotor activities (Cooper, In press). These observations indicate that the LP-pulvinar complex is, in some presently unknown fashion, linked to the subcortical components of the sensorimotor organization. Although pulvinar lesions in the intact primate are not associated with any detectable change in sensorimotor activities, Cooper's observations have their analogy in lesions to VL. Such lesions are ineffective in altering sensorimotor functioning in the intact primate, but are effective in favorably altering abnormal motor activities in the damaged human nervous system. Previous studies have demonstrated that activities arising in Cd, EP and MT are powerful determinants of activities in the corticospinal tract (Frigyesi, Purpura, 1964). The results here show that these basal ganglia and medial thalamic synaptic pathways generate effects in DLT neurons similar to those in the dorsal thalamic relays of the cerebello-corticospinal projection system. Thus data in the present report lend support to Dr. Cooper's proposition that LP-pulvinar complex is involved in the regulation of sensorimotor activities.

## ACKNOWLEDGEMENTS

This work was supported by a grant from the National Institute of Neurological Diseases and Stroke, NIH, NS

09898–02. The physiological data summarized in this paper were obtained in various collaborative studies carried out with J. Machek and A. Rabin. I am indebted to both of these colleagues for kindly permitting publication of data obtained in joint studies.

# References

Armengol, V. and Palestini, M.: Relationship between pulvinar and optic tract, lateral geniculate body and superior colliculus. *Acta. Neurol. Latinoamer. 14:*17–27, 1968.

Clüver, P.F. de V. and Campos-Ortega, J.A.: The cortical projection of the pulvinar in the cat. *J. Comp. Neurol. 137:*295–307, 1969.

Cooper, I.S.: The pulvinar and ventrolateral nucleus of the human thalamus. In: *Corticothalamic projections and sensorimotor activites.* Frigyesi, T.L., Rinvik, E. and Yahr, M.D. (Eds.). N.Y. Raven Press. In press.

Feldman, M.H. and Purpura, D.P.: Prolonged conductance increase in thalamic neurons during synchronizing inhibition. *Brain Res. 24:*329–332, 1970.

Frigyesi, T.L. and Machek, J.: Basal ganglia-diencephalon synaptic relations in the cat. I. An intracellular study of dorsal thalamic neurons during capsular and basal ganglia stimulation. *Brain Res. 20:*201–217, 1970.

Frigyesi, T.L. and Machek, J.: Basal ganglia-diencephalon synaptic relations in the cat. II. Intracellular recordings from dorsal thalamic neurons during low-frequency stimulation of the caudatothalamic projection systems and the nigrothalamic pathway. *Brain Res. 27:*59–78, 1971.

Frigyesi, T.L. and Purpura, D.P.: Caudate effects on evoked activity in nucleus ventralis lateralis. *Physiologist 6:*182, 1963.

Frigyesi, T.L. and Purpura, D.P.: Functional properties of synaptic pathways influencing transmission in the specific cerebello-thalamocortical projection system. *Exp. Neurol. 10:*305–324, 1964.

Frigyesi, T.L. and Rabin, A.: Basal ganglia-diencephalon synaptic relations in the cat. III. An intracellular study of ansa lenticularis, lenticular fasciculus and pallidosubthalamic projection activities. *Brain Res. 35:*67–78, 1971.

Godfrained, J.M., Meulders, M. and Veraart, C.: Visual receptive fields of neurons in pulvinar, nucleus lateralis posterior and nucleus suprageniculatus thalami of the cat. *Brain Res. 15:*552–555, 1969.

Mettler, F.A.: *Neuroanatomy.* St. Louis, Mosby, 1948.

Palestini, M., Borlone, M. and Tejos, E.: Electrophysiological study of the relationship between pulvinar and amygdala. *Acta Neurol. Latinoamer. 14:*92–98, 1968.

Purpura, D.P. and Cohen, B.: Intracellular recording from the thalamic neurons during recruiting responses. *J. Neurophysiol. 25:*621–635, 1962.

Purpura, D.P., Scarff, T. and McMurtry, J.G.: Intracellular study of inter-
nuclear inhibition in ventrolateral thalamic neurons. *J. Neurophysiol.*
28:487–496, 1965.

Siqueira, E.B.: The temporo-pulvinar connections in the Rhesus monkey.
*Arch. Neurol.* 13:321–330, 1965.

Simma, K.: Der Thalamus der Menschenaffen. *Psychiat. et Neurol.* (Basel)
134:145–175, 1957.

Walker, A.E.: Internal structure and afferent-efferent relations of the
thalamus. In *The Thalamus.* D.P. Purpura and M.D. Yahr (Eds.) N.Y.,
Columbia Univ. Press, pp. 1–12, 1966.

### DISCUSSION

**Dr. Van Buren:** I had wanted to ask Dr. Frigyesi about
the current levels he was employing in stimuli and how they
were applied and his anesthesia levels. I think the possibility
you bring up of the pathway is a very good one and I will
show it later I think, in man, coming in underneath the basal
ganglia. I don't have it going through because we are just
using myelin studies. As can be seen very clearly from the
myelin studies that is the pathway.

**Dr. Frigyesi:** We did not monitor levels of stimulating currents. The ways we distinguished between true entopeduncular evoked effects and spurious effects due to spread of
stimulating current to the internal capsule included control
preparations such as those with ablated sensorimotor cortex,
those with degenerated fibers of the pyramidal tract, or, during
stimulation the entopeduncular activities in the medullary
pyramidal tract were monitored. We used a variety of controls,
details of which have already been published (Frigyesi,
Machek, 1969). These procedures enabled us to distinguish
between effects in the thalamus which were related to activation of those axons which arise in entopeduncular nucleus
and those which were consequences of spread of stimulating
current to the axons of the internal capsule. At the present
time we are convinced that the thalamic effects, which I have
shown, are real effects from the entopeduncular nucleus and
not spurious effects due to inadvertant activation of a variety
of long axons traversing the internal capsule in ajuxta-

entopeduncular position. Regarding your second question, the cats were unanesthetized, encéphale isolé preparations, though local anesthesia was applied during surgery.

**Question from floor:** We have been placing lesions in the anterior suprasylvian gyrus of cats and young kittens and we found a large projection to LP and some to the pulvinar. But what is surprising is that especially in LP the projection appears to be bilateral and I was wondering if in the monkey you saw any evidence of projection to the pulvinar or LP from the contralateral hemisphere?

**Dr. Siqueira:** In our work fortunately we had a very large supply of animals and in general confined my lesions to one side and produced degeneration in one hemisphere. I have never found any evidence of a direct connection from one side to the other. Of course, the indirect connections, such as collaterals or multi-synaptic pathways I have not studied in these experiments, but as far as we can tell in the monkey, I do not see any evidence of bilateral representation. Even when, for instance, a total ablation of the cerebral hemisphere was done, the area of pulvinar was perfectly intact. Now what will happen when they do study these animals when there is very extensive ablation of the pulvinar, I don't know. This is still to be studied.

**Dr. Trachtenberg:** A question for Dr. Frigyesi and Dr. Siqueira: Dr. Frigyesi, could you in any way identify these pulvinar neurons you were studying, as to whether they are Golgi type I or Golgi type II cells?

**Dr. Frigyesi:** No, I cannot further identify them at this time.

**Dr. Trachtenberg:** Dr. Siqueira, in order to make your pulvinar lesions, did you cut the corpus callosum or did you retract it?

**Dr. Siqueira:** I retracted and at least in the frozen sections there was no evidence of lesions; but we did find some lesions on the corpus callosum. In other words in some animals there were lesions in the corpus callosum, and in some animals there weren't. Eventually, I hope to have a large population of animals in test and when these animals are eventually sacrificed, I hope to obtain some animals in which the corpus callosum was left intact despite the massive lesion in pulvinar bilaterally, because a lesion in the corpus callosum can vitiate and confuse the results.

**Dr. Trachtenberg:** I would just like to bring on a bit of controversy. I have made lesions in area 8 of the macaque brain, and find that there is a small but real area of degeneration in the medial part of the pulvinar. As we have only a few animals at this time, I cannot give you very much more detail.

**Dr. Poirier:** I would like to add something to the last comment. Using the osmic acid method we also disclosed a positive (black) reaction, in the lateral part of the pulvinar following temporal lobe lesion, as did Dr. Siqueira. But as mentioned earlier this morning, this area does not contain myelinated fibers so that we could not expect this intensely stained material to correspond with myelin degradation. It is also important to mention that we observe this osmic acid positive reaction only after a few weeks, and it may well correspond to a local reaction (glial?) associated with retrograde degeneration in this area of the pulvinar as a consequence of lesions of the temporal lobe.

**Dr. Siqueira:** In the first slide that I showed they were quite small. I am grateful that you brought this up. These particular lesions in the monkey were found within less than two weeks. Actually, most of these animals were waiting two weeks and on the actual nissl preparation there was no marked glial proliferation; I have seen this in many other preparations in which I used nissl preparations. This is not due to glial proliferation. Where this material came from I do not know; no one is clear. If you check the textbooks in histochemistry, it is interesting, really no one has a perfect explanation. But besides this, I would say that about half of my preparations do confirm the presence of this degeneration.

**Dr. Rakic:** I thought at this point we should bring up a question of the nucleus lateralis posterios (LP) which is quite appropriately included in the program of the symposium, but which has received very little discussion so far. Ann Graybiel in work now in progress in Dr. Nauta's laboratory at M.I.T., made lesions in LP in cats and found, rather interestingly, that the cortical area to which LP projects makes almost a semi-circle around the area of pulvinar and n. lateralis inter-medus (LI) projections. At the outer side it borders on the somesthetic, visual and auditory cortex (Fig. 16). Therefore, the area of cortex to which the pulvinar-LI projects is not in direct continuity with the primary sensory areas. Instead it is enclosed by the projection area from LP. I think that this finding fits rather well with the ontogenic and phylogene-tic developmental sequences of both posterior thalamus and parieto-temporo-occipital cortex. The association cortex develops between the primary projection areas. Apparently the cortex associated with LP develops first and then the cortex enclosed by it, associated with the pulvinar expands in parallel with enlargement of the pulvinar. Dr. Graybiel's work also suggests that the input to the LP-pulvinar complex have been less well known simply because it does not have

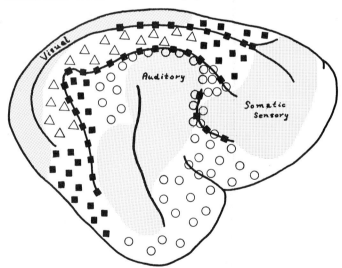

Figure 2–16. Schematic diagram of the cat's cerebral hemisphere which illustrates the major visual, auditory and somesthetic sensory areas (stippled) and the areas of neocortical fiber degeneration resulting from lesions of the lateralis posterior (solid squares), posterior nuclear group (open circles) and the pulvinar n. lateralis intermedius (triangles). Diagram courtesy of Dr. A. Graybiel (*Brain, Behavior and Evolution* 1972, 6:363–393).

a dense lemniscal input analogous to the projections to the ventrobasal complex or the geniculate bodies. Instead, she has demonstrated some degenerating fibers in the LP-pulvinar complex after various manipulations such as cordotomy, lesions in the inferior and superior colliculi, the pretectal region and the brainstem tegmentum. These data are consistent with the speculation that axons from many different brain structures converge towards the pulvinar-LP complex, but no single lesion produces a dramatic effect.

**Dr. Gilman:** I wish to ask Dr. Siqueira two questions. The first is related to the evidence he presented of connections between pulvinar and temporal lobe. Specifically, are there reciprocal temporal lobe projections to the pulvinar? My second question stems from your comment that there is some degeneration in the tectum of the brain stem after pulvinar lesions and yet all of the pulvinar cells degenerate after hemispherectomy. Is it possible that pulvinar cells bifurcate, sending one axon to the hemisphere and another axon to the tectum, and, if so, to which part of the tectum does the pulvinar project? These anatomical considerations may give important clues as to the mechanism of effect of pulvinar lesions in humans.

**Dr. Siqueira:** I must apologize again. Your second question is a result of my poor presentation—the lesions going to the tectum did not arise from the pulvinar. The degeneration as far as the tectum is concerned, is secondary to the lesions in the occipital cortex. If I implied that these arise from neurons from the pulvinar, I am sorry because that was not the case at all. And as far as the connections between the temporal lobe in the pulvinar itself, in my opinion, they are reciprocal. I believe there is a much heavier connection from the temporal lobe to the pulvinar than vice versa by the sheer number of neurons involved, but as I have demonstrated in some preparations the degenerating fibers seem to go either way when the monkey is sacrificed between two or three weeks.

**Dr. Gilman:** Dr. Van Buren, can you expand somewhat on the work you've doing on the chimpanzee?

**INVITED DISCUSSION**

## Anatomic Studies of Pulvinar in Humans
### J.M. VAN BUREN, M.D.

The work on the chimpanzee has not been related to the pulvinar directly—it is simply to redefine the site of architectural and tract relationships in the lateral ventral complex which I had spoken about as a preliminary paper in the Fulton Society this June. I am not really sure that I can add to the present discussion on the pulvinar, but I will be happy to tell you what little I know about it.

Our material consists of a series of serially sectioned human brains with paired sections at ten or twenty-section intervals stained for cells and myelin. Combining our modest resources with Dr. Yakovlev's extensive collection we have been able to prepare serial reconstructions of nearly 60 human brains with chronic destructive lesions (Van Buren and Borke, 1972). In this series, 28 brains showed degeneration in various segments of the pulvinar.

In regard to the question of frontal connections, I can only say that we found no evidence that lesions anterior to the central fissure result in retrograde cell loss in the pulvinar. A word of caution in this regard is in order, however. The posterior portion of n. medialis (n. medialis dorsalis) is myelin poor and the cells themselves closely resemble those of the adjacent pulvinar. This resemblance has caused some anatomists to classify the n. medialis and pulvinar together as a "fronto-parietal association nucleus". In man we have separated the two nuclei by arbitrarily connecting the scattered groups of intralaminar cells in this region and defining this as the frontier. In monkey, particularly in the transverse plane, this boundary may not be easy to define. Thus lesions in the posterosuperomedial frontal region (which lead to degeneration in the posterior pole of n. medialis) might be interpreted as causing cell loss in n. pulvinaris depending upon how the investigator draws his line of separation between the two nuclei.

Dr. Frigyesi's finding that firing patterns in the pulvinar

can be influenced by stimuli in the anterior half of the cerebrum is beyond comment by an anatomist. If I understand correctly, his latencies indicated a multisynaptic pathway. Anatomical degeneration studies are limited to discovering damage to the processes of the cell whose soma is under observation and possibly the next adjacent neuron in the stream (Van Buren 1963).

With regard to Dr. Siquira's study of the cerebrothalamic connections of the pulvinar, I would like to present three cases which may serve as examples to illustrate our conclusions about the connections of the pars oralis and pars medialis of the pulvinar. These segments were selected for brief presentation since there is little evidence of their connections in the literature.

The n. pulvinaris, pars oralis, is defined as the roughly conical anterior pole of the pulvinar which is thrust like a wedge between the posterolateral border of n. centralis (centre median) and the posteromedial border of n. ventrocaudalis (n. ventralis posterior). Its posterior border is taken as an arbitrary line joining the posterior poles of these two nuclei.

Six cases with relatively restricted cell loss in the pars oralis of the pulvinar lead us to conclude that this part of the nucleus had discrete connections with the region of the parietal operculum of the cerebral cortex.

Case LS LXXVIII (Fig. 17 and 18). This was an infarct of two years' duration which resulted in transient aphasia and weakness of the right arm.

The damage included the superior insula and lower postcentral gyrus (degeneration in the parvocellular portion of the n. ventrocaudalis), a small extension into the posterior transverse temporal gyrus (degeneration in the corpus geniculatum mediale) and cortical loss in the inferior third of the precentral gyrus and rolandic operculum (degeneration in n. lateropolaris, n. ventrooralis, internal and external segments, and n. medialis). In conjunction with the cases cited above, the cortical loss in the parietal operculum has been considered associated with the area of degeneration in the pars oralis of the pulvinar (sections L 1461 and L 1501).

# LS LXXVIII L

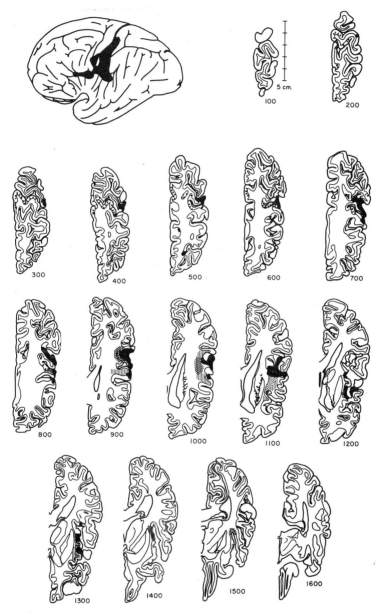

Figure 2–17. LS LXXVIII—an infarction of two years' duration. In this and subsequent diagrams, black areas = necrosis, vertical hatching = myelin loss, diagonal hatching = gliosis, horizontal hatching = cell loss. Small triangles in the cortex indicate Betz cells and the position of the precentral cortex.

# LS LXXVIII L

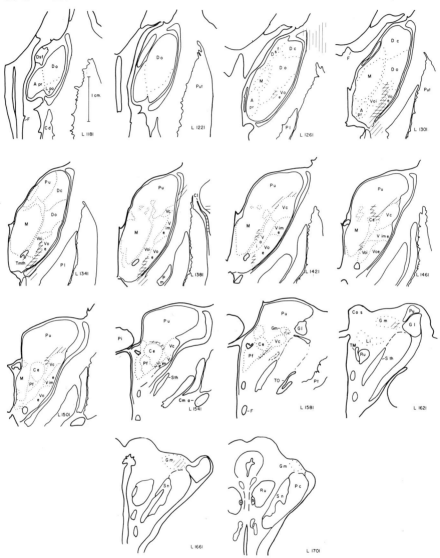

Figure 2–18. LS LXXVIII—thalamic reconstruction (cf. Fig. 1 for abbreviations).

The n. pulvinaris, pars medialis, has been defined as the medial portion of the nucleus which is largely free of the myelinated bundles characterizing the lateral half. The pars medialis extends posteriorly to include the posterior pole of the pulvinar.

Our evidence, although based upon ten cases, must be offered with some reservations since the lesions were of complex nature. In general, there seemed considerable evidence that the medial half of the pulvinar is related to the medial aspect of the parietal, temporal, and probably the anterior occipital regions. Lesions above the level of the splenium were accompanied by cell loss superiorly in the n. pulvinaris medialis while those below showed the cell loss inferiorly in the nucleus. The connections along the anteroposterior axis of the nucleus followed the anteroposterior axis of the medial hemisphere with the posterior pulvinar pole being connected to the region of the medial temporo-occipital junction.

Case A–64–96 (Fig. 19 and 20). This was an infarct of 13 months' duration apparently secondary to a period of hypertension during surgery. The lesion was limited to the cortex. On the medial aspect of the hemisphere it ran from the posterior frontal region nearly to the parieto-occipital fissure. It ran downward to involve the cingulate (limbic) gyrus largely in the posterior portion. It extended laterally from the midline about 2.5 cm. in the frontal region and somewhat further in the parietal area. Small superficial additional infarcts were present in the lateral occipital and frontal opercular regions.

In the pulvinar there was marked shrinkage and loss of the normally convex posterosuperomedial outline. The cell loss largely lay in the superior half of the medial part of the nucleus. The posterior pole was free of degeneration despite the loss in the occipital convexity. The spread of cell loss into the more lateral portion of the pulvinar (sections L 922, L 962) seemed related to the lateral spread of the infarct in the parietal region. Cell loss in the other nuclei seemed appropriate to the cortical destruction in the cingulate and lateral frontal regions.

A-64-96   L

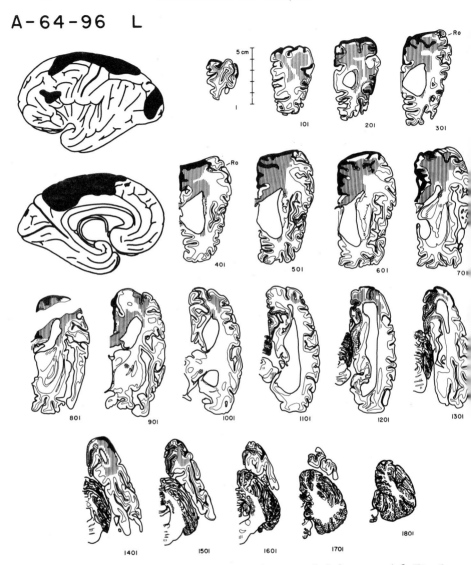

Figure 2–19. A–64–96—an infarction of 13 months' duration. (cf. Fig. 1 for abbreviations, in addition the primary visual cortex is indicated by hatching in the cortex which is perpendicular to the cortical surface).

# A – 6 4 – 96 L

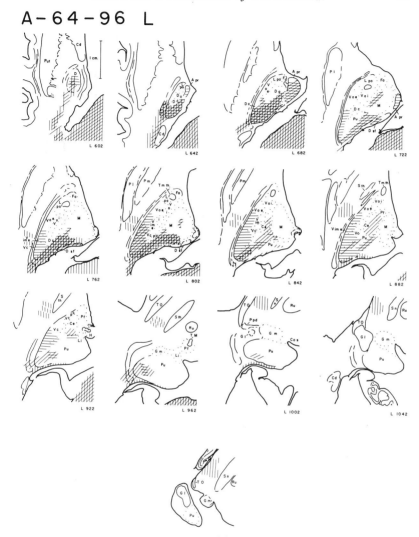

Figure 2–20. A–64–96—thalamic reconstruction (cf. Fig. 1 for abbreviations).

L LIV R

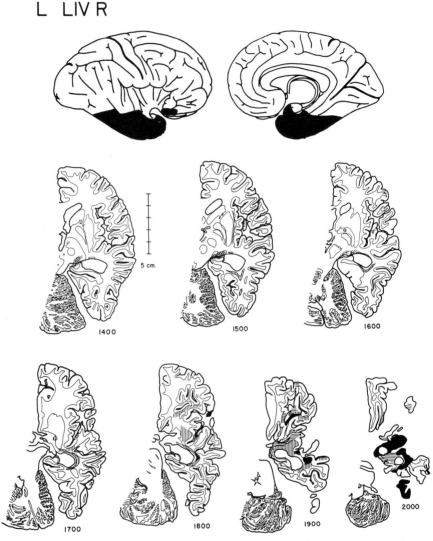

Figure 2–21. L LIV—a temporal lobectomy of two years' duration (cf. Fig. 1 for abbreviations).

Case L LIV (Fig. 21 and 22). This patient died two years following a temporal lobectomy for seizures. The surgical removal in the first temporal gyrus included the anterior half of the first transverse temporal gyrus. The removal extended

# L   LIV   R

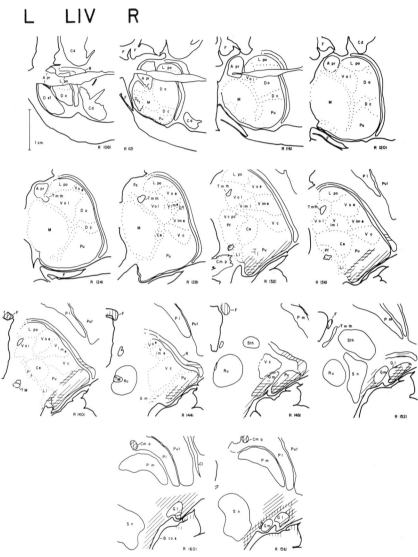

Figure  2–22. L LIV—thalamic reconstruction (cf. Fig. 1 for abbreviations).

downward from this point to include the other temporal gyri.
The pes hippocampus was damaged, and all but the posterior tip of the uncus and the superomedial amygdala removed. A small incidental lesion was present on the frontal
operculum.

The degeneration in the pars medialis of the pulvinar lay exclusively in the inferior part adjacent to the n. limitans. The more lateral extension of the degeneration in R 1361 was considered to be related to the posterolateral temporal removal. The interruption of the visual and auditory radiations produced the expected degeneration in the medial and lateral geniculate bodies.

## References

Van Buren, J.M.: Trans-synaptic retrograde degeneration in the visual system of primates. *J. Neurol. Neurosurg. Psychiat.* 26:402–409, 1963.
Van Buren, J.M. and Borke, R.C.: *The Nuclei and Cerebral Connections of the Human Thalamus.* Springer–Verlag, Heidelberg, Vol. 1. 1972.

## DISCUSSION

**Dr. Gilman:** I believe we face a problem in interpretation of the presented data. Dr. Van Buren has presented some very beautiful evidence demonstrating that the parietal lobe contributes to the pulvinar, and yet, Dr. Siqueira was unable to demonstrate connections between parietal lobe and pulvinar. I wonder if these two presentations could be brought together in some fashion by the presenters. Dr. Van Buren, do you think that the discrepancy results from the fact that you are studying humans and Dr. Siqueira is studying monkeys? Dr. Siqueira, do you believe that the problem has arisen because your lesions have not encroached sufficiently on the parieto-occipital region or upon the boundary zone? How are we to handle these conflicting data?

**Dr. Van Buren:** My personal view is that there is a very great difference of course between monkey and man's brains —I would hope so at least. We have to remember of course that the monkey has its primary visual cortex coming way out here, it's very close to the auditory relationship, indeed to the post central gyrus, a very small area here which could correspond I believe with the human association cortex, at least this would be my view. And possibly this association cortex just hasn't expanded medially in the monkey where we seem to find it in man. What is your view Dr. Siqueira?

**Dr. Siqueira:** I agree with Dr. Van Buren that there is of course a difference, but a medial primary projection should be found in both animals, and I believe that one of the explanations is the one that Dr. Van Buren has just given, that the visual cortex extends more laterally in monkeys than in humans. On the other hand, I don't have any animals in which a large lesion was in the posterior parietal lobe, so I believe we have two explanations. One is the difference in the animals and two is lack of lesions in the parietal lobe. I don't have any lesions in the medial aspect or the medial portion of the parietal lobe.

**Dr. Gilman:** If I recall correctly, Dr. Earl Walker studied the effects of cortical ablations in macaque monkeys many years ago and found degeneration in pulvinar following lesions of the boundary zone between parietal and occipital cortex.

**Dr. Siqueira:** Yes, you are correct, it was in his 1938 textbook.

**Dr. Gilman:** If I could clarify this issue further, I believe that your present findings are in conflict with the traditional view, based upon Walker's work, which indicated that the pulvinar projects to parieto-occipital cortex and not solely to the temporal lobe.

**Dr. Siqueira:** I have often wondered why Walker *et al.* hadn't studied the pulvinar and that was one of the main reasons I was studying the temporal lobe, and there was a large discrepancy between my work and Walker's 1938 textbook, in that he emphasized that the connection is between the temporal lobe and the pulvinar—mainly the posterior portion of the temporal lobe. That's why I went into all this; probably because I found this discrepancy. It is difficult to explain. Even recently there has been a textbook showing that there is a projection from the optic nerve to the pulvinar. In some of our animals I also carried out studies in which a lesion was placed in the optic nerve, but could not find any connection between the pulvinar and the optic nerve.

**Dr. Trachtenberg:** It seems that we're getting into the question of the pulvinar. Although I don't propose to be an expert on this matter, I would like to summarize some recent literature on the subject. In addition to the work that you have already mentioned, there is of course the classic study of Chow (1954) in which he reports retrograde degeneration in pulvinar after lesions of parietal, temporal, or occipital cortices. This was followed by the retrograde degeneration studies of Locke (1960) which demonstrated degeneration in the pulvinar from lesions in the temporal pole. In addition to this there are three more recent papers that should probably be brought to the fore. One is by Wilson and Cragg (1967) on the macaque; they showed that area 17 does not project to the pulvinar. In 1971, Spatz, Tigges and Tigges experimenting on the squirrel monkey report that there is a very small projection from area 17, particularly from layers 5 and 6, which projects to the pulvinar. In addition to these there is the paper by Cragg and Ainsworth (1969) which shows that areas 18 and 19 project to the pulvinar; they accept Wilson and Cragg's data at face value. Insofar as subcortical connections are concerned, this too is an area of conflict. Campos-Ortega *et al.* (1970) report degeneration in the pulvinar in the macaque and baboon after lesion of the optic nerve. And I have injected trineated leucine into the eye of the macaque and find, using autoradiographic techniques, silver grains in the pulvinar in the same area as Campos-Ortega *et al.* I should caution that both my preliminary findings and data of Campos-Ortega *et al.* are derived from parasagittally sectioned material. Nuclear boundaries are often difficult to assess in such material. To go much further would get us into very much of the old literature which, because of the techniques used, may be incomplete or that Papez (1939) had reported connections from dorsalis medialis to the pulvinar.

## References

Andersen, P. and Andersson, S.A.: *Physiological Basis of the Alpha Rhythm.* New York, Appleton-Century-Crofts, 1968.
Andersen, P., Andersson, S.A., and Lomo, T.: Nature of thalamo-cortical relations during spontaneous barbiturate spindle activity. *J. Physiol.* (London) *192:*283–307, 1967.

Andersson, S.A., Holmgren, E., and Manson, J.R.: Synchronization and desynchronization in the thalamus of the unanesthetized decorticate cat. *Electroenceph. Clin. Neurophysiol. 31*:335–346, 1971.

Andersson, S.A., Holmgren, E., and Manson, J.R.: Localized thalamic rhythmicity induced by spinal and cortical lesions. *Electroenceph. Clin. Neurophysiol. 31*:347–353, 1971.

Andersson, S.A. and Manson, J.R.: Rhythmic activity in the thalamus of the unanesthetized decorticate cat. *Electroenceph. Clin. Neurophysiol. 31*:21–34, 1971.

Campos-Ortega, J.A., Hayhow, W.R., and Clüver, P.F. de V.: A note on the problem of retinal projections to the inferior pulvinar nucleus of primates. *Brain Res. 22:* 126–130, 1970.

Chow, K.L.: A retrograde cell degeneration study of the cortical projection field of the pulvinar in the monkey. *J. Comp. Neurol. 93:* 313–340, 1950.

Cragg, B.G. and Ainsworth, A.: The topography of the afferent projections of the circumstriate visual cortex of the monkey studies by the Nauta method. *Vision Res. 9:*733–747, 1969.

Locke, S.: The projection of the medial pulvinar of the macaque. *J. Comp. Neurol. 115:*55–170, 1960.

Papez, J.W.: Connection of the pulvinar. *Arch Neurol. Psychiat. 41:*277–289, 1939.

Pollen, D.A. and Trachtenberg, M.C.: Some problems of occipital alpha block in man. *Brain Res. 41:*303–314, 1972.

Spatz, W.B., Tigges, J., and Tigges, M.: Subcortical projections, cortical associations, and some intrinsic intralaminar connections of the striate cortex in the squirrel monkey (Samiri). *J. Comp. Neurol. 140:*155–173, 1970.

Wilson, M.E. and Cragg, B.G.: Projections of the lateral geniculate nucleus in the cat and monkey. *J. Anat.* (London), *101:*677–692, 1967.

# CHAPTER 3

# THE ROLE OF THE THALAMIC PULVINAR-LP COMPLEX IN MODULATING NEOCORTICAL REACTIVITY

E. Crighel, M.D. and A. Kreindler, M.D.

THE FUNCTIONAL SIGNIFICANCE of the Pulvinar-Lateralis Posterior Complex (Pul-LP) in the cat is still little understood. The anatomical data concerning the Pul-LP connections with cortical areas and with subcortical structures, on the one hand, are of a controversial nature, and, on the other hand, are insufficient to understand the functional role of the complex. The physiological data are equally controversial. Some, (Buser *et al.* 1959) suggest that the Pul-LP complex would act as relay nuclei for responses evoked in neocortical association areas, while others (Bignall *et al.* 1966, 1964) seem to disprove it.

In previous investigations (1968) we demonstrated that visual, auditory and somesthetic inputs are projected to the Pul-LP complex. At some points we found a monosensory, while at others a polysensory projection. We also detected some deaf points where no projection from the periphery occurred. In the polysensory points the conditional stimulus induced occlusion and enhancing mechanisms. Electrical shocks to the Pul-LP complex evoked responses with short latencies not only in the association areas of the neocortex, but also in the primary projection areas, except the somesthetic ones. The flash-responsive points in Pul-LP complex project either to the visual, to the association, or to the auditory areas of the neocortex, indiscriminately, or to the auditory and association only. The same phenomenon was seen with the Pul-LP points of auditory or somesthetic projection. This was called the commutation function of the Pul-LP complex. This phenomenon was particularly conspicuous for the somesthetic points in Pul-LP, which never project to the somesthetic neocortical areas. There was also Pul-LP projection to contralateral neocortex, through the opposite Pul-LP complex, via the massa intermedia. The contralateral responses showed a different recovery cycle, and persisted after homolateral neocortical depression, elicited after KCL application; the responses evoked contralaterally in the Pul-LP by electrical shocks to the Pul-LP complex, were shorter in latency than those evoked in the contralateral neocortex.

The polysensory convergency, the occlusion and facilitation phenomena, the commutation function, as well as the dispersion of inputs towards large homo and hetero lateral neocortical areas, enabled us to consider this complex as a sensory integrating structure. These results agree with those of Hotta and Terashima (1965), Hirata *et al.* (1967), Palestini and Guzman (1966).

Very little has been said about the influence of Pul-LP on neocortical reactivity. Battersby and Oesterreich (1963), Brown and Marco (1967) showed that tetanization of the dorsal region of the pulvinar elicited a posttetanic enhancement of visual evoked responses, especially in the posterior marginal gyrus, only ipsilateral to the pulvinar stimulated. Long (1959), Morillo (1961), Hotta and Terashima (1965), and Hirata *et al.* (1967), by stimulation or by lesion of the Pul-LP complex, also found some evidence concerning the influence of the Pul-LP complex on the visual cortex and the lateral geniculate body. The present investigation represents a systematic study of the influence of the Pul-LP complex on the neocortical reactivity to peripheral (visual) and central [lateral geniculate body (GL) and Pul-LP] stimuli.

## MATERIAL AND METHOD

Experiments were performed on 58 adult cats. For tracheotomy and mounting in the stereotaxic apparatus the animals were anesthetized with ether. The cats were immobilized by gallamine triethiodide (Flaxedil[R] ), injected periodically and the respiration was maintained artificially. Craniotomy was performed and the brain was exposed under local anesthesia with 1 percent novocaine. All the other sites of incision (for tracheotomy, denudation of the veins) and the pressure points of the stereotaxic apparatus, were also infiltrated with 1 percent novocaine. The animals were maintained, during the experiment, in a dark room, with constant temperature at 35°C ± 2°C and constant humidity. The experiment started 1 hour after cessation of ether anesthesia.

The electrocorticogram (ECoG) was recorded monopolarly (reference electrode on the occipital bone) by means of silver-silver chloride ball electrodes. The deep electrodes used for recording and stimulation were either of Bronk Type (two stainless insulated wires in a needle; the non-insulated tips were at 0.3–0.4 mm distance), or concentric electrodes (the distance between the noninsulated tip of the central electrode and the noninsulated ring of the external electrode being 1 mm). From the thalamic GL (lateral geniculate body), Pul, and LP nuclei, the records were only bipolar. The electrodes were stereotaxically introduced, according to the atlas of Jasper and Ajmone Marsan. During the experiment the electrode location was physiologically checked. After the experiment the location was anatomically checked, using Nissl's and Spielmeyer's staining methods. For visual stimulation bright white flashes (0.125, 0.25 and 0.5 J intensities) delivered by a photostimulator, were used. The bulb of the photostimulator was 50 cm in front of the cat's eyes. The pupils were dilated by atropine. Each bulb discharge was accompanied by a very slight click. For electrical stimulation of the thalamic nuclei, rectangular pulses, 0.15 ms width, at liminal, subliminal and slightly supraliminal intensities, were used. The thalamic nuclei were repetitively stimulated at low frequencies (6–10 cycles/sec, or with 100 cycles/sec, for tetanic stimulation. High frequency stimulation lasted 50–300 msec, and preceded by 25–350 msec the peripheral stimulus. The responses were registered on a cathode-ray oscilloscope, with the spot divided by an electronic switch. R-C coupled amplifiers with symmetrical input, 0.1 sec time constant, as well as a frequency up to 2 K cycles/sec were used. Single or superimposed sweeps were photographed. A statistical evaluation was also made.

## RESULTS

Between the 6th and the 9th frontal planes, 44 points of the Pul-LP complex were investigated. Only 16 of the 44 points when stimulated with 100 c/s, for various durations of the bursts of stimuli and with different stimulus intensities, did not change the neocortical reactivity to peripheral stimuli. Five of the inactive points were situated in n. suprageniculatum or in its vicinity and the others were very rostrally or caudally (F: 8.5–9 or F: 6–6.5). The other Pul-LP points showed a more or less marked influence on the neocortical reactivity when tetanically stimulated. It is noteworthy that not all the active points had a similar influence on the reactivity of the neocortex to peripheral stimuli, which appears from the following:

(a) Liminal or slightly subliminal tetanization of some points of the Pul-LP complex enhanced the visual responses only in the homolateral marginal gyrus (Fig. 1). It is of note that in the same figure the point situated near the suprageniculate nucleus failed to change (after the tetanization) the neocortical reactivity. Other points such as point 2 in figure 2, showed a post-tetanic influence not only in the homolateral visual area, but also on the suprasylvian gyrus, while post-tetanization of point 3 in the same figure (Fig. 2) exerted a post-tetanic enhancement of visual responses in both visual areas, homo and hetero laterally. The enhancement sometimes involved only the initial components of the responses to flashes, (Fig. 2, point 2), or the late slow component (Fig. 1, point 2). The differences seen after tetanization were statistically significant.

(b) The changes in neocortical reactivity to peripheral stimuli (flashes) depended on the intensity of the stimuli and the total duration of the burst of stimuli utilized for the Pul-LP

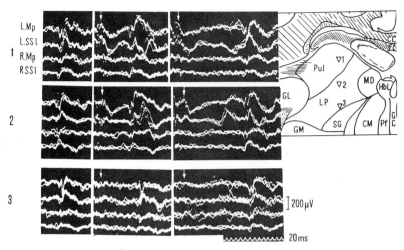

Figure 3–1. Tetanization of three points in the pulvinar-lateralis posterior complex (Pul-LP). Arrows indicate the end of tetanization which lasted 50 ms. The first column of photos represents the controls. The tetanization of points 1 and 2 enhance the visual evoked responses only in homolateral posterior marginal gyrus. The tetanization of point 3 failed to modify the neocortical reactivity to flashes. Abbreviations: L = left. R = right. Mp = posterior marginal gyrus. SSL = lateral part of the suprasylvian gyrus.

stimulation. Figure 3 shows a tetanization with 2.5V which lasted 50 msec with an enhancing effect on the visual responses in both visual areas (homo and hetero laterally) only at short delays between the end of the tetanization and the visual stimulus; with long delays only a homo lateral enhancement was seen. The tetanization of the LP point elicited an afterdischarge in the homolateral suprasylvian gyrus and therefore it was impossible to be certain about the action on the flash-evoked responses in this area. A longer duration of the tetanization (100 ms) modified the reactivity to flashes in the homolateral visual area (only at short delays) and in the homolateral suprasylvian gyrus and thereafter no influence was seen with this duration of the tetanic bursts on the marginal gyrus either homo or contra-laterally. The tetanization with 200 ms. elicited only a homolateral suprasylvian enhancement. The 100 and 200 msec tetanization did not elicit an afterdischarge in suprasylvian gyrus. Weak intensities of tetanization (0.9V) elicited a substantial afterdis-

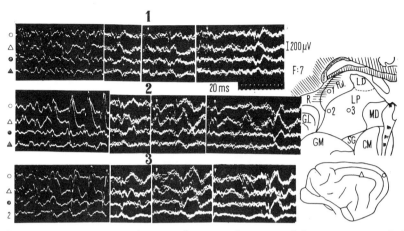

Figure 3–2. Tetanizing bursts of 50 ms duration of three points in left Pul-LP. Arrows indicate the end of tetanization. Tetanization of point 1 fails to modify the neocortical reactivity. Tetanizations of point 2 enhance the responses in posterior marginal gyrus, as well as in the suprasylvian gyrus, only homolaterally. Tetanizations of point 3 enhance the flash evoked responses in both marginal gyri (homolaterally and contralaterally to the LP stimulation. In range 3 is a registration from point 2 of LP. No change in flash evoked responses in point 2 was seen after tetanization of point 3. The first column of photos show incremental responses elicited in the neocortex by low rate stimulations of the Pul-LP points. The dark signs indicate the site of the neocortical registration points contralaterally to the Pul-LP stimulated.

charge in the homolateral suprasylvian gyrus and induced an enhancement of the visual responses only in the homolateral marginal gyrus, when the tetanization lasted 200 msec.

(c) The enhancement was like a post-tetanic action because it appeared only 25–30 msec after the cessation of the tetanic burst of stimuli. Slow rate of stimulation (6–10 cycle/sec) which elicited incremental responses, did not modify the neocortical reactivity. (Fig. 4).

(d) No essential changes were seen at GL (Fig. 5) and LP levels (Fig. 2) after the tetanization of Pul-LP. The responses to flashes in GL showed, in some cases, very few changes, (a lengthening of the slow phase, as in Fig. 3).

(e) The geniculo-cortical responses did not undergo changes after tetanization of Pul-LP; slow rate stimulation

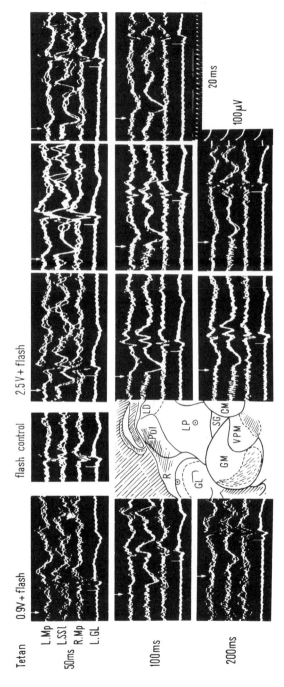

Figure 3–3. Tetanization of a point in the left LP with two intensities and different durations of the tetanizing bursts. Arrows indicate the end of tetanization. See detailed explanation in text. Abbreviations as in Fig. 1. GL = lateral geniculate body.

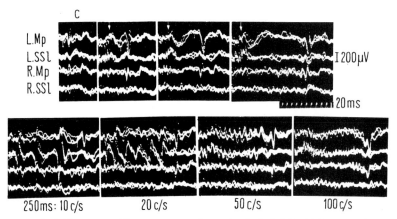

Figure 3–4. First row: Tetanization of a point in left LP elicits an enhancement of the flash evoked responses in homolateral Mp. only at short delays between the end of the tetanization (indicated by arrows) and the flash delivering. Second row: Low rate stimulations (10 cps) do not modify the flash evoked responses. Same abbreviations as in Fig. 1. C = control.

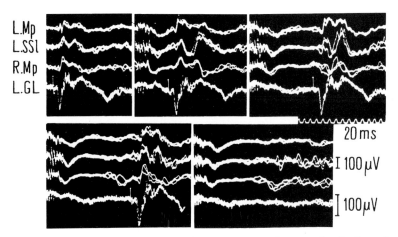

Figure 3–5. Tetanization of a point in the left LP enhances the flash evoked responses in both Mp, and in homolateral SSP. No change in the responses to flashes in GL. Abbreviations as in the previous figures. The first photo segment is control for flash evoked responses. The last photo segment for tetanization only.

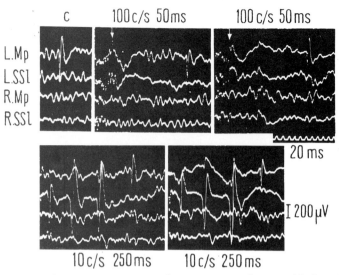

Figure 3–6. Either tetanization or slow rate stimulation of left pul does not change the geniculo-cortical responses. Abbreviations as in the previous figures.

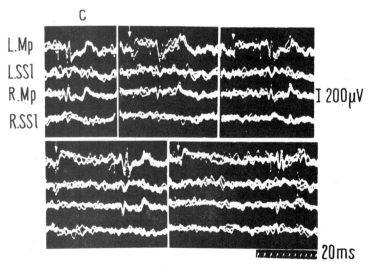

Figure 3–7. Tetanization with liminal intensity, 100 c/s, 50 ms duration to the left lateral geniculate body does not modify the neocortical reactivity. The same abbreviations as in the previous figures.

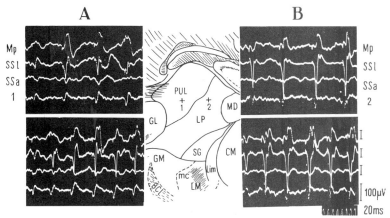

Figure 3–8. A. The stimulation of point 2 (in LP) elicits a positive-negative response in point 1 (in pul). Repetitive stimulation with 6 or 10 c/s in point 2 elicits incremental responses in point 1 in homolateral SSL (augmenting type) and in homolateral Mp (recruiting type).

B. Stimulation in point 1 and registration in point 2 and in the same neocortical areas as in A. In point 2 there are no obvious responses; in the neocortical points there are augmenting and recruiting responses. Abbreviations: Mp = posterior marginal gyrus. SSL = lateral part of suprasylvian gyrus; SSA = anterior part of the suprasylvian gyrus.

of the Pul-LP did not bring about any change either (Fig. 6).

(f) Tetanization of the relay nuclei of the thalamus (GL) failed to cause any posttetanic change in the reactivity to peripheral stimuli of the visual area (Fig. 7).

(g) No modifications were seen in the EEG tracings after tetanization of Pul-LP with the above mentioned parameters. Liminal electrical shocks to a point of Pul-LP complex of the thalamus sometimes elicited responses in another point of the same complex. These responses were positive-negative in size, with 1.5–3 msec latencies. Slow rate repetitive stimulations (6–10 cycle/sec) elicited incremental responses of the augmenting type in the Pul-LP point where the responses were registered. No correlation could be found between the incremental responses elicited in the neocortex and those elicited in Pul-LP. Between the two investigated points of the Pul-LP complex there was generally a one-way connection. (Fig. 8).

## DISCUSSION

From our previous investigations it appeared that the Pul-LP complex in the cat is, from the physiological point of view, a nonhomogeneous structure, with an integrating function. This complex projects not only homolaterally but also to the contralateral neocortex. The present investigations confirm these conclusions and permit further considerations concerning the function of the Pul-LP. The most pertinent point here is the enhancement of the flash evoked responses in the neocortex which appears after Pul-LP tetanization, like a post-tetanic effect. Our results agree only partially with those of Battersby and Oesterreich (1963) and Brown and Marco (1967), because of the differences in the experimental conditions. Our results showed that this enhancing action was exerted not only homolaterally and almost exclusively on the posterior marginal gyrus, but also contralaterally and also on the suprasylvian gyrus. One should note that not all the investigated points had the same effect; some points only had a restricted homolateral influence, while some had a widespread influence, both homo- and contralaterally. This is in agreement with the view that functionally the Pul-LP complex is not a homogeneous structure. From our results we could not infer any topographical organization of the functional differences. The responses elicited in the Pul-LP by single and slow rate repetitive stimulations of other points of the same complex indicated that in spite of the lack of homogeneity of the structure, there are interrelations between the various compartments of the Pul-LP. We have not tested the influence of Pul-LP tetanization on the excitability of the motor area. Kogan, discussing our paper presented at the Havana symposium on Cortico-subcortical relationships, mentioned that he had found changes in the excitability of the motor neocortex after tetanization of Pul-LP complex with 50 cycle/sec. All these investigations suggest that the Pul-LP comples, particularly some structures of this large complex, which should be closely investigated, can be considered as a modulator of the neocortical reactivity and excitability.

One should also note that the post-tetanic action on the

neocortical reactivity, was dependent on the intensity and especially on the duration of the burst of tetanizing stimuli. Short bursts, which generally enhanced the responses to peripheral stimuli at the neocortical level, may thus be considered to have an excitatory action, while long lasting bursts elicit a depression. The appearance of afterdischarges only after short bursts of Pul-LP tetanizations, support this point of view. We consider, however, this explanation to be insufficient. The correlation between the duration of the bursts of Pul-LP tetanic stimulation and the "post-tetanic" action is not only quantitative: as was shown in Fig. 3, the neocortical area involved in the post-tetanic action also depends on the duration of tetanization. It may be that depending on the "quantity of energy" utilized for Pul-LP stimulation, different pathways are used: some pathways are blocked, other permeabilized, etc. We have not sufficient data yet to support this point of view, but we consider that we can explain in the same manner the fact that in some cases the initial components of the responses to peripheral stimuli are enhanced, while in others only the late slow components are enhanced. The post-tetanic action has no relation whatever with the incremental responses elicited by slow rate stimulation of the Pul-LP complex, which did not influence the neocortical reactivity. We feel that different pathways are involved and also different mechanisms are put into action. The reactivity changes to peripheral stimuli elicited by Pul-LP tetanization seems to take place at the neocortical level. As already mentioned above, the responses in lateral geniculate body or in Pul-LP elicited by peripheral stimuli were not at all or only very slightly modified by Pul-LP tetanization. It seems very hard to explain the mechanisms involved in this action at the neocortical level, bearing in mind also that the geniculo-cortical responses were not modified by the same type of Pul-LP stimulation. A general action via diffuse projecting nuclei of the thalamus (in yet unpublished investigations we found physiological evidence for the existence of such pathways), or via colliculus superior-MRF (Crighel and

Kreindler, 1969, Armengol and Palestini and co-workers), Hirata and co-workers (1967) etc. is difficult to accept as the EEG pattern remained unchanged after Pul-LP tetanization.

Our present experiments suggest that the Pul-LP, apart from its integrating function can also be included among the complex of structures involved in the modulating activity of the neocortical reactivity.

## REFERENCES

Armengol, V., and Palestini, M.: Análisis electrofisilógico de algunas conexiones del pulvinar. *VI Congreso de la Asociación Latinoamericana de Ciencias Fisiologicas.* Vina del Mar, Chile, p. 29, 1964.

Battersby, W.G., and Oesterreich, R.E.: Neural limitations of visual excitability. IV photic enhancement following lateral thalamic stimulation. *Electroenceph. Clin. Neurophysiol.* 15:849–863, 1963.

Bignal, K.E.: Comparison of optic afferents to primary visual and polysensory areas of cat neocortex. *Exp. Neurol.* 17:327–343, 1967.

Bignal, K.E., Imbert, M., and Buser, P.: Optic projections to nonvisual cortex of the cat. *J. Neurophysiol.* 29:396–409, 1966.

Brown, T.S. and Marco, L.A.: Effects of stimulation of the superior colliculus and lateral thalamus on visual evoked responses. *Electroenceph. Clin. Neurophysiol.* 22:150–158, 1967.

Buser, P., Borenstein, P., and Bruner, J.: Etude des systèmes "associatifs" visuels et auditifs chez le chat anesthesié au chloralose. *Electroenceph. Clin. Neurophysiol.,* 11:305–324, 1959.

Crighel, E. and Kreindler, A.: Relations between the Pulvinar-Lateralis posterior complex and the collicular region in cat. *Rev. Roum. Neurol.* 6:273–277, 1969.

Hirata, U., Fuse, Sh., and Koikegami, H.: Studies on the paralimbic brain structures. II. Experiments on the Pulvinar nucleus of the cat. *Acta Med. et Biol.* 15:113–129, 1967.

Hotta, T. and Terashima, S.: Audio visual interaction and its correlation with cortical stimulation in the lateral thalamus. *Exp. Neurol.* 12:146–158, 1965.

Kreindler, A., Crighel, E. and Marinchescu, C.: Neocortical excitability and relationships with the Pulvinar-Lateralis posterior complex. in: *Cortico-subcortical relationship in sensory regulation.* (D. Gonzalex Martin, ed.) Havana, *Acad. Sci.* 75–84, 1966.

Kreindler, A., Crighel, E. and Marinchescu, C.: Integrative activity of the thalamic Pulvinar-Lateralis posterior complex and interrelations with the neocortex. *Exp. Neurol.* 22:423–435, 1968.

Long, R.C.: Modifications of sensory mechanisms by subcortical structures. *J. Neurophysiol.* 22:412–427, 1959.

Morillo, A.: Microelectrode analysis of some functional characteristics and interrelationships of specific, association and non-specific thalamo-cortical system. *Electroenceph. Clin. Neurophysiol. 13:*9–20, 1961.

Palestini, M., and Guzman, S.: Electrical activity of the pulvinar related to sleep and wakefulness in cat. in: *Cortico-subcortical relationship in sensory regulation.* (Ed. D. Gonzalez-Martin) Havana, *Acad. Sci.* 313–325, 1966.

Palestini, M., Barlone, M., and Tejos, E.: Electrophysiological study of the relationship between pulvinar and amygdala. *Acta Neurol. Latinoamer. 14:*92–98, 1968.

## DISCUSSION

**Dr. Frigyesi:** Were you able to elicit an evoked potential in pulvinar by a shock to the hind leg?

**Dr. Crighel:** The shock to the hind paw elicited a response only in the lateralis posterior complex and not in the pulvinar.

**Dr. Trachtenberg:** Since you have told us of a contralateral cortical influence of the pulvinar, have you tried stimulating in one pulvinar or one LP and recording in the other? And have you considered any possible pathway aside from callosum of course which might mediate this contralateral response?

**Dr. Crighel:** In our previous investigations (1966, 1968) we showed that an electric shock in LP elicited a response in the contralateral LP. In some cases it doesn't elicit any response in the contralateral neocortical area while in other cases it also elicited a response in the contralateral neocortical area but the neocortical responses had longer latencies than those in the contralateral LP complex.

**Dr. Poirier:** I think there is one point that will be raised quite often in this discussion: it is the fact that the pulvinar is crossed by important fiber bundles that are represented by cortico-tectal and cortico-tegmental tracts which, at least to some extent, have a bilateral projection in the brain stem, as demonstrated by Henderson and Crosby. I think that in any experiment involving stimulation one must take account that these groups of fibers which do not originate in the pulvinar may be stimulated.

**Dr. Crighel:** In all our experiments we considered this possibility but we studied primarily the LP nucleus where there are less passage fibers than in pulvinar. We stimulated 44 points and we got different types of influences and I think that it is impossible that in all the points with bilateral influence only passage fibers were stimulated. Brown and Marcos (1967) and Kreindler and Crighel (1970)* showed that the tegmental and pretegmental regions had depressing action on the visual areas and not an enhancing one on the Pulvinar-LP complex.

**Dr. Frigyesi:** I didn't quite understand your interpretation of this finding. Was it post-tetanic potentiation or depression and at which site? Are you implying that you observed facilitatory and inhibitory after effects at the two recording sites? The importance here is that the kind of mechanism you propose bears on the issue of how the pulvinar is actually connected to the other parts of the sensori-motor organization.

**Dr. Crighel:** It is very difficult to explain our findings. As was shown, it was an enhancing effect on responses to peripheral stimuli at neocortical level only. No changes in thalamo-cortical potentials or in the responses evoked by peripheral stimuli at the GL or LP level were seen. Therefore we consider that Battersby and Oesterreich's and Brown and Marco's interpretation that it is a post-tetanic effect is too simple. I think that this modulating effect of neocortical reactivity, exercised by the Pulvinar-LP complex involves in its mechanism some other structures also which we were not yet able to make evident.

---

* Kreindler, A. and Crighel, E., Collicular influences on the thalamo-cortical association and the primary visual projection systems in cat. *Rev. Roum. Neurol.* 7:275–281, 1970.

**CHAPTER 4**

# SENSORY FUNCTION OF THE PULVINAR*

D. E. RICHARDSON, B.S., M.D., F.A.C.S.**

## INTRODUCTION

**M**Y INTEREST in the sensory function of the pulvinar initially stemmed from clinical studies with lesions placed
in the area of the intralamina nuclei of the thalamus to prevent
chronic pain. The lesions were primarily placed in the area
of the centre median and were not always effective, as the
relief of pain was sometimes short in duration. In an attempt
to improve the relief of pain, the lesions were gradually moved
posteriorly from the centre median to involve the medial pulvinar. The lesions in the pulvinar were made in twelve
patients and produced significant relief of chronic pain similar
to that found with lesions in the area of the centre median
nucleus (Richardson, 1967).

The clinical picture following lesions of the medial pulvinar
is one of relief of chronic pain, but preservation of acute
pain. The postoperative sensory examination indicates that
vibratory sensation, pinprick, position sense, and light touch
remained clinically intact, while chronically induced pain
such as that from bone invasion by tumors is dramatically
relieved. The patients have very little in the way of mental
changes, euphoria, frontal lobe signs, or changes in personality to indicate the effect is similar to that produced by frontal
lobotomy or limbic system changes. The duration of pain
relief is similar to that found in the more anterior lesions

* Supported by The Cancer Association of Greater New Orleans.
** Associate Professor of Neurological Surgery, Department of Surgery, Division
of Neurosurgery, Tulane University Medical School, New Orleans, Louisiana.

and the sensory control or relief of pain lasts for approximately four to six months when the pain sometimes returns. In addition to this, acute exacerbation of pain such as pathological fracture or a fall involving the pre-existing area of pain has produced an acute return of pain.

This phenomenon of pain relief following medial pulvinar lesions could not be explained on the basis of its anatomical connections as described in the literature. Anatomical studies indicated that the main afferent influx into the pulvinar stems from the parietal lobe.

Walker (1938), using Nissl and Marchitechniques, found only connections to the cortex. Anderson and Berry (1959), Mehler, Feferman, and Nauta (1960), and Mehler (1966), using the Nauta-Gygax staining technique for unmyellinated fibers and preterminals found evidence of sensory fiber termination in the intralamina nuclei, ventral posterior medialis and lateralis, reticular formation, and tegmentum, but none in the pulvinar following cordotomy.

Electrophysiological studies by Kruger and Albe-Fessard (1960), Rose and Mountcastle (1952), and Rose and Woolsey (1958) have shown activation of cells in the ventrobasilar complex (including VPM and VPL) as well as portions of the ventrolateral nucleus, centre median, parafascicularis, and posterior complex (magno-cellular medial geniculate body and nucleus posterior). However, studies of the pulvinar, anterior nuclei group, and nucleus medialis dorsalis were conspicuously lacking in activation by sensory input.

The goal of this work is to achieve a better understanding of the role of pulvinar in pain processing, and to take a fresh look at its anatomical connections and its functional role in light of the results obtained with lesions in human patients. Electrophysiological techniques were chosen for this work because it was felt that anatomical degenerative studies might lead to incomplete findings; the pathways to the pulvinar, like those projecting to other paleospinothalamic centers, are most likely polysynaptic via the reticular formation, and would require careful functional dissection in order to map them out.

A number of approaches were utilized to achieve the above goal, including recording of gross potentials and single cell responses to peripheral input. These experiments were carried out both in the intact animal and in animals lesioned or transected in various parts of the neuraxis; this latter method was used to determine the routes by which information reached the pulvinar, and the role played by various structures in the modulation of responding in that structure.

## METHODS

One hundred cats were used for the basic physiological studies of the sensory function of the pulvinar. Ninety subjects were employed in the evoked potential work and 10 in the micro-electrode studies. The technique for preparation of the animals and recording techniques have been previously described (Richardson, 1970), but, in brief, consist of anesthetizing the animal with ether anesthesia, performing a tracheostomy, a left femoral venotomy, and a right femoral arteriotomy for cannulation to allow measurement of blood pressure and administration of fluids and drugs. The incision sites, scalp, and ear canals are infiltrated with 1% Xylocaine® throughout the experiment. The calvarium is exposed by a scalp incision in a well anesthetized scalp and appropriate removal of the skull carried out to allow stereotactic electrode implantation. The right sciatic nerve is exposed in the upper thigh to allow stimulation with bipolar stimulation electrodes. Cordotomy, stimulation, and recordings from the spinal cord are carried out by exposing the cord in the mid-dorsal area by laminectomy. The animal is allowed to reach consciousness to the point of the onset of voluntary muscular movement and D-Tubocurarine is injected intravenously in small doses to prevent motor activity and allow studies to be carried out in the unanesthetized animal. Artificial respiration is induced and $CO_2$ levels in the expired air are monitored. The temperature is measured by a rectal thermometer and maintained with a heat lamp and circulating hot water pad during experiments. Skin electrodes are made from small Michel clips and attached to the face or hind limb when necessary. Recordings

are made with bipolar 0.5 mm silver-silverchloride ball electrodes  separated by 1 mm intervals. Some recordings were
made by silver plated steel electrodes separated by 1 mm
at the tip.

Electrodes are implanted in the cat brain in the appropriate
areas using the atlas of Juan Jimenez-Costalleno (1949) and
stimulation of the skin or sciatic nerve carried out by a Grass
stimulator at 45 volts, 0.5 msec duration for skin stimulation
and 30 volts, 0.2 msec duration for sciatic nerve stimulation.
In most of the macro-electrode experiments, 50–100 stimuli
were summed by the use of an Enhancetron 1024 computer
to allow averaging of the signal and extract the signals from
background noise. Recordings of the traces were made with
Tektronix high gain differential preamplifier and 564 scope
and recorded on a polaroid trace recording camera.

Identical technique for preparation of the animals was used
in the single cell studies, except that recordings were made
through glass micro-electrode pipettes drawn to a tip diameter
of a 2–4 micra and filled with 2 molar sodium chloride.

Lesions were made by radiofrequency current from a Grass
radiofrequency lesion maker that had been precalibrated in
cat brains. Confirmation of electrode position was done by
fixation of the entire head and staining with cresyl violet
after sectioning.


## RESULTS

### A. Gross Potentials

Evoked responses were easily obtained in the area of the
pulvinar from either skin stimulation or stimulation of the
sciatic nerve. As can be see from Figure 1, the evoked
response is a complex potential with a number of components.
In an effort to determine the source of the various components
and the pain pathway leading to the pulvinar, transections
and/or lesions were performed at various levels of the
neuraxis. Further, the modulation by the pulvinar of other
structures involved in pain processing was also investigated.

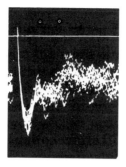

Evoked response in the

contralateral pulvinar from

facial stimulation.

20 msec/div. 20 responses.

Cat 40-1

Figure 4–1. Twenty superimposed recordings from the pulvinar of the cat evoked by contralateral stimulation of the skin of the face. Trace duration 200 msec., cat TP–40.

## *a. Spinal Paths*

The question arises as to whether the impulses to the pulvinar travel in the dorsal column or the ventral lateral column. Sensory evoked responses were recorded before and after bilateral dorsal column section or ventral lateral cordotomy in the upper dorsal cord. Figure 2 shows a reduction of the evoked response by approximately 75% after bilateral dorsal cordotomy. This result is parallel to changes seen by Shafron and Collins (1964) in the centre median. It is to be noted that ventralis posterior lateralis (VPL) responses are totally abolished after a dorsal cordotomy as can be seen in Figure 3.

Presumably, dorsal cordotomy abolishes a large amount of the sensory input to the pulvinar, except for pain and temperature. Under these conditions, a mapping of the pulvinar was performed with computer-averaged evoked responses. Figure 4 shows such a map with 1 mm off-set passage, and using 1 mm bipolar electrodes. In spite of some variation in configuration it can be seen that the responses remain

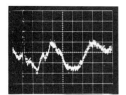 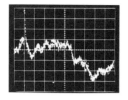 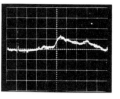

Evoked response in left pulvi-    ...after dorsal column section.    ...after bilateral mesencephalic
nar to right leg stimulation...                                        reticular formation lesion

25 msec / div                        100 responses

TP 93 - pl - 1 - 8 - 14

Figure 4–2. Effect of dorsal column section alone and in combination with mesencephalic reticular formation lesions on evoked responses in the pulvinar. The left tracing is the evoked response in the pulvinar from sciatic nerve stimulation in the intact animal. The middle tracing is following dorsal column section and reveals abolition of the primary positive and negative component and a marked enlargement of the late large positive wave, indicating an increase in the late component. However, following bilateral mesencephalic reticular formation lesion, marked reduction of the volume of the response and phase reversal is noted. It was found on anatomical confirmation studies that the reticular formation had been incompletely destroyed and probably resulted in some retention of the evoked response in the late phase. One hundred averaged responses per tracing, 150 msec per tracing, cat TP–93.

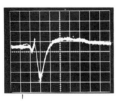 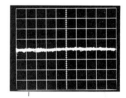

PRE-CORDOTOMY                        POST-DORSAL CORDOTOMY

EFFECT of DORSAL COLUMN SECTION

Recording from ventral posterior lateral thalamus

AP = + 9.5; Lat. = 7; Ht. = 0        10 msec / cm        50 µv / cm

Right leg stimulation        Cat SI # 19 (2 - 5)

Figure 4–3. Recording from the ventral posterior lateralis nucleus of the thalamus before and after section of the dorsal columns. Complete abolition of the evoked response in the primary sensory nucleus of the thalamus following dorsal cord section indicating little or no evoked response traversing the spinothalamic tract, per se. 100 msec per tracing, cat SI–19.

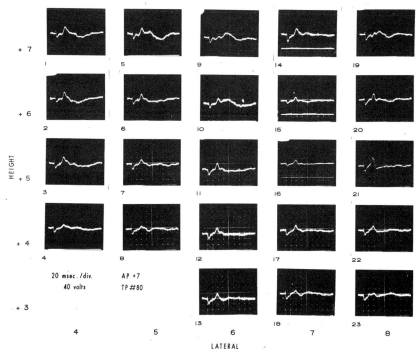

Figure 4–4. Mapping of the evoked responses in the pulvinar in the frontal projection after dorsal cordotomy utilizing computer averaging of 100 responses per tracing to eliminate background noise. Orientation is given in Horsley-Clark coordinates. 200 msec per tracing, cat TP–80.

very similar throughout the area of study, which involved 4 × 5 mm frontal planes through the main mass of the pulvinar.

On the other hand, bilateral ventrolateral cordotomy caused a reduction of the primary response evoked in the pulvinar with some apparent enhancement of the secondary component as demonstrated in Figure 5.

## b. Reticular Formation

Previous studies have indicated both anatomically and physiologically that the sensory impulses reaching the centre median were from the reticular formation (Mehler, 1966; Shafron and Collins, 1964). This was tested by recording evoked responses in the pulvinar and producing lesions in the

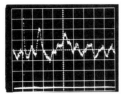
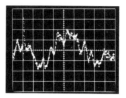

Evoked response in contralateral
pulvinar to ® leg stimulation
prior to anterolateral cordotomy.

25 msec. / div.      100 responses
                        averaged

Evoked response in contralateral
pulvinar to ® leg stimulation
after bilateral anterolateral cordotomy.

25 msec. / div.      100 responses
                        averaged

TP  Cat # 88

Figure 4–5. Average recording of 100 responses from the pulvinar of the cat to sciatic nerve stimulation. The left illustration is the response with an intact spinal cord, and the right response is following bilateral antero-lateral cordotomy. The configuration of the evoked response has been altered, plus there is enhancement of the late component of the evoked response. 100 average responses, 250 msec per trace, cat TP–88.

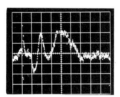

Evoked response in left pulvinar
to right leg stimulation...

...after bilateral mesencephalic
reticulum formation lesion

25 msec / div      100 responses

TP # 90    8 - 15

Figure 4–6. Effect of mesencephalic reticular formation lesions on evoked responses in the pulvinar. The left tracing is an evoked response in the pulvinar from sciatic nerve stimulation in the intact animal. The right tracing is the same evoked response after bilateral coagulation of the mesencephalic reticular formation. The evoked response has been changed primarily by modification of the late component, abolition of the large negative wave, and replacement by much smaller alternating negative and positive wave. This would tend to indicate that the primary contribution of the mesencephalic reticular formation to the evoked response is through a multisynaptic late component. 100 averaged responses per tracing, 250 msec per tracing, cat TP–90.

reticular formation at the level of the mesencephalon. It is interesting that the sensory input to the pulvinar is obviously carried both by dorsal and ventral lateral columns, and that complete ablation of sensory evoked responses in the pulvinar could not be obtained without doing both a dorsal cordotomy and a reticular formation lesion. Figure 6 reveals modification of sensory input into the pulvinar by bilateral mesencephalic reticular formation lesion, but that near complete ablation of the evoked response could only be obtained by a combination of dorsal cordotomy and bilateral reticular formation lesions as in Figure 2. This leads to the assumption that dorsal column pathways do not traverse the reticular formation exclusively to reach the pulvinar, but that ventral lateral spinothalamic tract pathways do.

### c. *Thalamic Nuclei*

It was possible that the sensory input to the pulvinar could arrive via the main sensory relay nucleus of the thalamus, the nucleus ventralis posterior lateralis. However, when coagulation of this nucleus was performed, the evoked response in the pulvinar remained essentially unchanged (Figure 7).

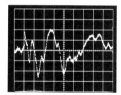    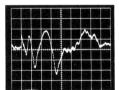

Evoked response in left pulvi-          ... after left VPL lesion.
nar to right leg stimulation...

             25 msec / div          100 responses

TP # 94     PL 4-6

Figure 4–7. Effect of lesions of the VPL on pulvinar evoked responses. The left tracing is the evoked response from sciatic nerve stimulation in the contralateral pulvinar. The right tracing is the same evoked response after lesioning the VPL nucleus of the thalamus. The pattern and volume of the evoked response is essentially unchanged following destruction of the primary relay nucleus of the thalamus.

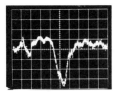
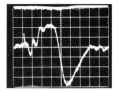

Evoked response in left pulvi-          ...after left CM lesion.
nar to right leg stimulation...

25 msec /div          100 responses'
TP 94 - 5 - 10

Figure 4–8. Effect of lesions of the centre median nucleus on evoked responses in the pulvinar. The left tracing is 100 averaged responses from the pulvinar and the tracing on the right is the experiment repeated after radiofrequency destruction of the centre median nucleus. It shows some enhancement of the evoked response, but no change in pattern and no dramatic modification of the components, except for some increase in volume. 100 averaged responses per tracing, 250 msec per tracing, cat TP–94.

The relationship of the centre median to the pulvinar was of interest because of the similarity in clinical response of patients with lesions in both of these areas. It was noted that the pathway of sensory impulses reaching the pulvinar might well be through the centre median nucleus since it does have connections to almost all of the other

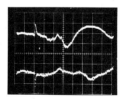

Top tracing: Sensory cortex.

Bottom tracing: Pulvinar.

Stimulation of sciatic nerve.

250 responses          5 msec/cm

Cat SI  #62-10

Figure 4–9. The top tracing is evoked response in the sensory cortex and the bottom tracing the evoked response in the pulvinar following contra-lateral sciatic nerve stimulation. The evoked response in the cortex and the pulvinar while different in configuration, are almost identical in time in relation to the stimulus artifact. 250 averaged responses, 50 msec per trace, cat SI–62.

thalamic nuclei (Walker, 1938). When lesions were made in the centre median and recordings made before and after from the medial pulvinar, enhancement of the evoked response in the pulvinar was seen after these lesions (Figure 8).

### d. Interaction with Cortex

The previously suggested function of the pulvinar as a sustaining nucleus of the parietal cortex led us to investigate the interplay between cortex and pulvinar in the processing of sensory phenomena. The possibility remained that sensory evoked responses in the pulvinar could be recurrent phenomena from the cortex which receives sensory input from VPL; however, it was made unlikely by the finding that VPL lesions did not significantly alter the responses in the pulvinar. Attempts to confirm this by cortical ablation and pulvinar recordings were unsuccessful in our hands due to difficulty in placing the electrodes in the appropriate areas of the pulvinar after the cortex was surgically removed. However, simultaneous recordings from the cortex and pulvinar were made, showing that the pulvinar response is almost identical in time to the cortical response to sensory input

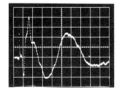    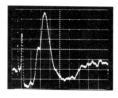

Evoked response in left parietal cortex from right leg stimulation...

...after left pulvinar lesion.

50 msec/div     100 responses
TP   94

Figure 4–10. Modification of cortical evoked responses by lesions of the pulvinar. The left response is the cortical evoked response from sensory input with an intact pulvinar and the right illustrates the alteration of the evoked response following electro coagulation of the ipsilateral pulvinar. The primary component has been shortened in duration and shortened in latency. The secondary component has been markedly enhanced in voltage and shortened in time duration. 100 averaged evoked responses, 500 msec per trace, cat TP–94.

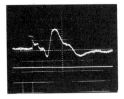 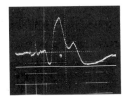 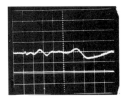

Leg stimulation alone    Pre-stimulation to pulvinar    Stimulation to pulvinar alone

Left intercallicular tegmentum

recording - right hind leg

100 averaged responses    stimulation.    10 msec/div

SI 10

Figure 4–11. Effect of the pulvinar stimulation upon evoked responses in the mesencephalic reticular formation. The left tracing is evoked response in the intercollicular tegmental reticular formation from sciatic nerve stimulation alone. The center tracing is with pre-stimulation of the pulvinar showing an enhancement of the evoked response. The third tracing shows the evoked response in the reticular formation from stimulation of the pulvinar alone, showing that the enhancement of the evoked response shown in the middle figure is not related to an additive effect. 100 averaged responses per tracing, 100 msec per tracing, cat SI–10.

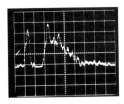 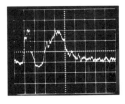 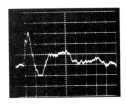

Evoked response in left    ...after lesion in pulvinar.    ...after lesion in centrum

intercallicular tegmentum    median.

from right leg stimulation...

50 msec / div    100 responses averaged

SI 17

Figure 4–12. Effects of lesions of the paleospinothalamic system on the mesencephalic reticular formation. The left illustration is the evoked response in the brain stem reticular formation in the intact animal. Following lesions of the pulvinar, the secondary component of the evoked response is reduced in volume and duration. Following addition of the lesion to the centre median, this late component of the evoked response is markedly reduced as compared to the baseline recording. 100 averaged responses, 500 msec per tracing, cat SI–17.

(Figure 9). Further, cortical responses were modified by lesions of the pulvinar as shown in Figure 10. Thus, the last two findings confirm the existence of the close interaction between cortex and pulvinar suggested by anatomical studies.

*e. Some Output Pathways*

Aside from its effect on cortex, the role of pulvinar activation in modifying responses in pain-related areas was studied. Prestimulation of the pulvinar increased evoked responses in the mesencephalic reticular formation as seen in Figure 11. On the other hand, lesions of the pulvinar caused a small decrease in these evoked responses. However, a marked suppression of reticular activation is obtained when centre median lesion was added, as noted in the study in Figure 12.

The reverse effect is noted with lesions in the VPL, a portion of the neospinothalamic pathway; such lesions led to enhanced responses in reticular pathways at the level of the mesencephalic reticular formation (Figure 13).

## B. Micro-electrode Studies

In an attempt to clarify the complicated evoked responses in the pulvinar to sensory input, extracellular micro-electrode recordings of single cell responses to sensory input were carried out in 10 cats.

Sciatic nerve stimulation and recordings from the pulvinar of extracellular cell firing patterns revealed that there are two types of cells that respond to sensory input. The Type I cell is a pulvinar cell that has a resting firing pattern of short bursts at infrequent intervals. With sciatic nerve stimulation of single shocks, this cell has a marked increase in firing rate following a latency of approximately 50 msec and lasting from 100 to 200 msec (Figure 14). If a Type I cell is presented with a burst of sciatic nerve stimulation lasting 3 seconds, they respond by a prolonged period of excitation and rapid firing lasting up to 6 minutes. Figure 15 shows the resting firing pattern and the response to a burst of sciatic nerve stimulation with prolonged rapid firing of the cell.

The second type of cellular response is noted in the pulvinar Type II cells that are markedly inhibited by sciatic nerve

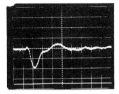

Before VPL lesion.

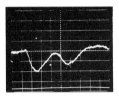

After VPL lesion. Sciatic
nerve stimulation. Recording
from tegmental reticular
formation.
Cat SI 33-7-12

Figure 4–13. Effects of VPL lesions on evoked responses in the reticular formation. The top response is a baseline recording made from the brain stem reticular formation evoked by sciatic nerve stimulation in the intact animal. The bottom response is the same recording following a destruction of the VPL by electrocoagulation. The changes induced by VPL lesion involve some phase reversal of the late component with increase in volume. 100 averaged responses, 50 msec per tracing, cat SI–33.

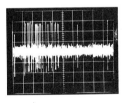

PULVINAR: TYPE I CELL RESPONSE
Response to single shock to
sciatic nerve.
Cat SI 68-2          50 msec/cm
Stimulation at 10 msec

Figure 4–14. Microelectrode recording of Type I cell response in the pulvinar to single shocks of the sciatic nerve showing activation of Type I cell with latency of approximately 50 msec and duration of firing of approximately 150 msec. 500 msec trace duration, cat SI–68.

PULVINAR TYPE I CELL RESPONSE

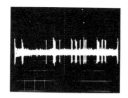

Resting firing pattern.

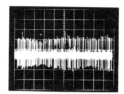

Following burst stimulation to
sciatic nerve.
Cat SI 72-9-11   500 msec/cm

Figure 4–15. Type I pulvinar cell showing basic resting firing pattern in the top illustration and marked activation by 3 second burst stimulation to the sciatic nerve. The duration of repetitive firing lasted approximately 6 minutes. Trace duration 5 minutes, cat SI–72.

stimulation. Figure 16 shows the Type II cell's response to single shocks of the sciatic nerve by prolonged period of inhibition lasting approximately 45 msec followed by a short period of increased firing and then a resumption of baseline firing rate. In response to burst stimulation of the sciatic nerve,

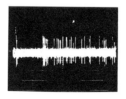

PULVINAR:
TYPE II CELL RESPONSE
Single stimulus to sciatic nerve-
(10 responses)      20 msec/cm
Cat SI-70-10

Figure 4–16. Pulvinar Type II cell showing 50 msec inhibition of cell firing by single shocks of the sciatic nerve. 200 msec trace duration, cat SI–70.

PULVINAR: TYPE II CELL RESPONSE

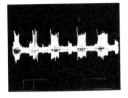

Resting   pattern.

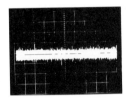

Following  burst  stimulation  to
sciatic   nerve.
Cat SI 73-9-10        1 sec /cm

Figure 4–17. Type II cell in the pulvinar showing the basic slow bursting repetitive firing pattern in the top illustration and complete abolition of firing following burst stimulation of the sciatic nerve in the bottom illustration, inhibition lasted 6 minutes. Trace duration 10 seconds, cat SI–73.

this cell responds by prolonged inhibition lasting up to 6 minutes. Figure 17 shows the resting repetitive bursting firing rate of the Type II cell and then its complete inhibition of firing following a 3 second burst of repetitive stimuli to the sciatic nerve.

## DISCUSSION

My initial studies in the human during thalamic operations for intractable pain has confirmed the contention of Bishop that there are in actuality two complete sensory systems (Bishop, 1958). The neospinothalamic system mediates epicritic or acute sensation primarily through the ventral posterior nuclei of the thalamus and the paleospinothalamic system, a multisynaptic pathway, through the reticular formation as seen in lower animals. My clinical studies have shown that the pathway through the centre median and medial pulvinar carries chronic pain or what has been called protopathic pain which co-exists with the more direct pathway mediating acute or epicritic pain. This double pathway was graphically demonstrated by a patient that had a centre median and pulvinar lesion made for relief of the chronic pain of cancer. Following his operation he received an acute burn of the forearm and hand that became ignited while filling a cigarette lighter. The patient had pain for approximately 3 minutes following which he had little or no pain and required no pain medication for the initial dressing or multiple dressing changes later for his second degree burns. This has also been tested by using a timed, high intensity heat light source for quantitating pain measurements before and after centre median or pulvinar lesions (Richardson, 1967). The threshold for acute epicritic pain does not change from before to after the operation which relieved the patient's chronic pain completely, and accurate localization was still found on pinprick testing.

In order to determine whether the medial pulvinar played a primary part in transmission of pain impulses, or whether it only modulated the pain pathway through facilitation, a series of studies was undertaken with local anesthesia, utilizing cats. They have revealed that the pulvinar is highly responsive to sensory input, including noxious stimuli. Further, the pulvinar appeared to receive its input directly from the reticular formation rather than being modulated by thalamic nuclei, such as VLP or centre median. A series of transaction studies led to the following conclusions. The major portion of the sensory input to the medial pulvinar is from the dorsal column, and might not involve pain. However, a significant portion, up to 25% of the response obtained by macro-electrodes, is due to ventral lateral column input.

Lesions of the reticular formation markedly reduce input to the pulvinar, however, such a lesion associated with a section of the dorsal columns almost completely abolishes evoked responses in the pulvinar, indicating that the primary small fiber input is through the reticular formation, as is the case for centre median.

Interestingly enough, stimulation of the pulvinar seems to enhance reticular formation sensory responses, but lesions of the pulvinar do not seem to dramatically reduce these responses. Yet, lesions of the centre median seem to reduce the activation of the mesencephalic reticular formation by sensory input probably due to a loss of some tonic descending facilitation. Lesions of the ventral posterior nucleus cause activation of the evoked responses in the reticular formation and seem to indicate that the neospinothalamic system has an inhibitory function in relation to the paleospinothalamic system. This does not seem surprising since the same phenomenon has been reported by Melzack and Wall in the spinal cord (Melzack and Wall, 1965).

Micro-electrode recordings have revealed two types of responsive cells, one responding by a prolonged period of silence after sciatic nerve stimulation, and the other with a prolonged period of firing following that same stimulation. This reciprocal cell reaction is obviously produced by activation of one cell and inhibition of the other. Although there does not seem to be any easy way to attribute to these cells a specific role in the gross potential, their response patterns remain interesting and can shed light on the functional significance of the pulvinar. Thus, these cells possess patterns not characteristic of simple transmission neurons, but probably related to inhibitory and facilatory roles—they exhibit long latencies and prolonged firing rates. Such a response pattern is consonant with their hypothesized role in processing chronic, long lasting pain. Further, these cells, as reported by Yoshi (1970), appear to respond to a variety of sensory inputs such as light touch, proprioception, and pinching of the skin; this responsiveness to multiple sensory input is characteristic of a number of structures involved in the transmission and modulation of pain, such as the reticular formation and centre median (Kruger and Albe-Fessard, 1960; Shafron and Collins, 1964).

It seems clear from the above findings that the pulvinar is intimately involved in pain processing; its function is modulated by a number of inputs classically associated with sensation; in its turn it is capable of modifying responsiveness in other structures processing noxious input.

## SUMMARY

Clinical studies in the human being indicate that the pulvinar is involved in the perception of chronic pain sensation and that chronic pain can be abolished by making lesions in the medial pulvinar as well as the centre median nucleus of the thalamus. Studies of evoked responses in the pulvinar of the cat reveal that evoked responses can be easily recorded from cutaneous or peripheral nerve stimulation and that these impulses to a large part are carried by the dorsal column and by a small part of the ventral lateral portion of the cord, probably the spinoreticular pathway.

Impulses thought to represent pathways for pain apparently reach the pulvinar through the reticular formation and are not abolished by lesions of the centre median. Single cell recordings from the pulvinar reveal two types by sensory responses, cell Type I that is markedly activated by sensory input with prolonged firing rates lasting up to 6 minutes and cell Type II that is markedly inhibited by sensory input for up to 6 minutes. The pulvinar appears to have more primary functions than sustaining the parietal cortex in its relation to sensation.

* Acknowledgment: I would like to thank Dr. Huda Akil for help in preparing this manuscript.

## References

Anderson, F.D. and Berry, C.M.: Degeneration studies of long ascending fiber systems in the cat brain stem. *J. Comp. Neurol.* 111:195–229, 1959.

Bishop, G.H.: The relationship between nerve fiber size and sensory modality; phylogenetic implication of afferent innervation of cortex. *J. Neurol. Ment. Dis.* 128:89–114, 1958.

Jimenez-Costalleno, J.: Thalamus of the cat in Horsley-Clark coordinates. *J. Comp. Neurol.* 91:307–330, 1949.

Kruger, L. and Albe-Fessard, D.: Distribution of responses to somatic afferent stimuli in the diencephalon of the cat under chloralose anesthesia. *Exp. Neurol.* 2:442–467, 1960.

Mehler, W.R.: The posterior thalamic region in man. *Confin. Neurol.* 27:18–29, 1966.

Mehler, W.R., Feferman, M.D., and Nauta, W.J.H.: Ascending axon degeneration following an anterolateral cordotomy in the monkey. *Brain,* 83:718–750, 1960.

Melzack, R. and Wall, P.D.: Pain mechanism: A new theory. *Science* 150:971–979, 1965.

Richardson, D.E.: Thalamotomy for intractable pain. *Confin. Neurol.* 29:139, 1967.

Richardson, D.E.: Differentiation of touch-proprioception and pain-temperature evoked responses in the mesencaphalon. *Current Topics in Surgery Research*, 2:197–204. New York, Academic Press, 1970.

Richardson, D.E.: Sensory function of the pulvinar. *Confina. Neurol.* 32:165–173, 1970.

Rose, J.E. and Mountcastle, J.B.: The thalamic tactile region in rabbit and cat. *J. Comp. Neurol.* 97:441–490, 1952.

Rose, J.E. and Woolsey, C.N.: *Biological and biochemical basis of behavior.* University of Wisconsin, 1958, pp. 127–150.

Shafron, M. and Collins, W.F.: Ascending spinal pathway of centre median nucleus in the cat. *J. Neurosurg.* 21:874–879, 1964.

Walker, A.E.: *The Primate Thalamus.* Chicago, University of Chicago Press, pp. 317, 1938.

Yoshii, N.: In discussion of: Richardson, D.E. Sensory function of the pulvinar. *Confina. Neurol.* 32:165–173, 1970.

## DISCUSSION

**Dr. Van Buren:** I'm interested in the coordinate to the centers of your lesions and how you used your lesions. Are you using then contralaterally or are you using them simultaneously, bilaterally? How? And approximately the size of your lesions?

**Dr. Richardson:** We have made lesions in multiple areas both unilaterally and bilaterally. The patients mentioned in this presentation have had lesions in either the centre median or pulvinar, or a combination of both, usually on opposite sides. Our coordinates are: centre median Fp = 10, Lat = 10, Ht = 0; Pulvinar Lp = 15–20, Lat = 10–15, Ht = 0–+10. Lesion size was 8 to 12 mm—diameter.

**Dr. Cooper:** I wonder if we could, before we continue this discussion, ask Dr. Waltz to very briefly summarize the cases from our service undergoing cryopulvinectomy who had pain in addition to the motor disturbance. These results confirm your own, and then we can go on with the discussion of the sensory functions.

## INVITED DISCUSSION
### DR. J. M. WALTZ

Our experience with pulvinectomy in the treatment of chronic pain has been limited to 14 cases. However, even with this small series of cases the results initially seem to indicate that this is an approach to the treatment of chronic pain. Our series included seven cases of dyskinesia. These patients' initial complaints were not those of pain. However, pain was of severe nature in these patients insofar as they were totally incapacitated by these painful spasms of the neck in the cases of torticollis and of the extremities in the cases of dystonia muculorum deformans. In these seven cases, six were totally relieved of their painful spasms and one case was relieved for one month and then spasms recurred. There were two cases of metatastatic carcinoma; in one case pain was unrelieved by cordotomy. It was subsequently relieved by a pulvinectomy. There was an additional case of metastatic carcinoma relieved for six months. There was one case of cerebral palsy with a spastic hemiparesis and corticoathetosis who had what we believed to be an arthritic pain condition of the right knee, which was relieved by pulvinectomy. There was one case with chronic low back pain, sciatica, that had been unresponsive to multiple fusions, and cordotomy. She initially was relieved but pain recurred in two months.

We have also had three cases of CNS lesions where we were not quite sure of the exact location of pathology or etiologic factors, but all had severe burning dysesthetic pain over one side of the body, or limited to the face and were totally relieved of the pain. Of these 14 cases, 11 were totally relieved of pain, approximately 79% of the group. Three of the cases recurred after temporarily being relieved.

The last case was a 24-year-old cerebral palsy victim who had been well compensated, was attending school until six years ago, when she developed a progressive pain-like syndrome over the left side of her body including her face. She had been worked up extensively at several institutions neurologically. All of these tests were negative. She was requiring approximately 50 mg. of Demerol every six hours to relieve her pain. Following a pulvinectomy she remained pain free. So at the present time we feel that in the long run the surgery is effective.

**Dr. Cooper:** Dr. Richardson's paper has confirmed the immediate alleviation of the painful experience without producing any sensory abnormality. It is a very important contribution. Kudo *et al.,* as you know, in Japan, have reported an extensive series of procedures, with relief of pain lasting in some cases one or two years. Our own work has only had short term follow-up. Dr. Richardson indicates that many of his cases have recurred. On the other hand, as an insight into the elaboration of pain, this is a very new and important advance, particularly as it is related to the recent work in the posterior column.

**Question from floor:** In regard to those patients who have recurred, how many lesions were you placing?

**Dr. Richardson:** Most of my patients have had simple unilateral medial pulvinar lesions in an attempt to keep the procedure as "clean" physiologically as possible. I have done bilateral pulvinar lesions and pulvinar lesions combined with centre median lesions for bilateral pain and in an attempt to prolong the pain relief with equivocal results as far as duration of relief is concerned. My best duration of relief is somewhat over a year, but many of my patients die from cancer, limiting the followup.

**Dr. Waltz:** We are making a medial lateral lesion.

**Dr. Richardson:** I think this would add more destruction to the pulvinar. I had not made a lateral lesion because of concern over difficulties reported with speech.

**Dr. Waltz:** This is part of the problem.

**Dr. Richardson:** Apparently this is not as much of a problem as I had thought. The problem now is to destroy as much of the sensory pulvinar as possible. I might even add a centre median lesion to it in an attempt to destroy a larger portion of this pathway.

**Dr. Frigeysi:** Inasmuch as the pulvinar is regarded as a component of the central motor organization, it is expected that a long fiber system is carrying information from the periphery projects to the pulvinar. So in this frame of reference, Dr. Richardson's presentation is very important and bears on the central issue of this symposium, because he demonstrated that indeed such long tract systems elicit responses in the pulvinar. A curious feature of Dr. Richardson's detailed data is that two negatives were elicited in the pulvinar by peripheral stimulation. The longer latency negative wave was abolished by either a reticular or a CM lesion, yet the shorter latency negativity waves persisted under these conditions. It appears that the short latency negativity is not related to the generation of the long latency negativity. It also appears that these responses are induced through a different pathway. The first negative wave exhibited remarkably short 15 msec latencies. What do you think its trajectory is?

**Dr. Richardson:** I have thought about that a lot and my initial impression was that the initial short latency wave in the macro-electrode recordings is due to transmission through the dorsal columns by large myelinated fibers which have a much more rapid transmission time and that the late response is probably due to the multisynaptic pathway through the reticular formation. However, some of our macro-electrode data does not necessarily bear this out, as well as the fact that when micro-electrode recordings are made of single cell responses, one begins to understand the remarkable complexity of the response in these nuclei and it tended to make me reluctant to assign specific functional significance to different portions of the evoked response, as has been done by many physiologists in the past. Some objections to the interpretation of the pathway for different components of this response is also the fact that dorsal cordotomy does not necessarily abolish the initial rapid evoked response and making lesions in the VPL does not do away with this portion of response either.

It is my feeling at this time that in the cat there are no pain fibers traversing the VPL and that there probably are fibers carrying acute or epicritic pain traversing the VPL in the human. I think that there is much more basic research needed in this area and perhaps these controversies will stimulate other people to further investigations along these lines.

# CHAPTER 5

# PULVINAR CONTRIBUTION TO OCULOMOTOR AND CORTICAL EEG ACTIVITIES

M.C. Trachtenberg, Ph.D. and J. Siegfried, M.D.

## INTRODUCTION

THE PULVINAR is the latest of a series of brain loci in which lesions are being made for relief from intractable pain (Richardson, Zorub, 1970; Siegfried, In Press; Wilson, Cragg, 1967) and more recently for relief from spasticity (Cooper, Waltz, Amin and Fujita, 1971), yet the functions of this structure are enigmatic. The pulvinar—a diencephalic nucleus which arises, in part, from a telencephalic anlage (Rakic, Sidman, 1969)—sits astride the techtopetal output of the occipital cortices, the internal corticotectal tract. In turn, it sends fibers to the occipital and temporal corticies (Chow, 1950; Locke, 1960) and receives inputs from these cortical loci (Cragg, Ainsworth, 1969; Spatz, Tigges, Tigges, 1970; Whitlock, Nauta, 1956; Trachtenberg, Akert, unpublished data).

The occipital cortices show considerable alpha rhythm; so does the pulvinar (Albe-Fessard, Arfel, Guiot, Derome, Hertzog, Vourc, Brown, Aleonard, De Laherran, Trigo, 1966). Mulholland and his colleagues (Mulholland, 1969) suggest that the presence or absence of the cortical alpha rhythm is related to activation of the neartriad of accommodation, activation which likely involves the internal corticotectal tract. In light of these associative data we have examined the relationship of the pulvinar and cortical alpha rhythms and the effect of pulvinar stimulation on the cortical alpha rhythm as well as on oculomotor activity.

118

## METHODS AND MATERIALS

Subjects for this report are 15 neurosurgical patients, 8 male, 7 female, ranging in age from 50–62 years. Four patients received bilateral nucleus pulvinaris lesions, eleven received unilateral nucleus ventralis lateralis thalamus lesions; the latter for relief of extrapyramidal motor disorders. One patient was anesthetized (pentrane, 0.3%), all other patients received only local anesthesia (procaine 5%) at pressure points and wound edges. All patients were subjected to a pneumoencephalogram before being physiologically studied.

Scalp EEGs were recorded by means of needle electrodes located according to the system of Hess (Fig. 4) while deep activity was recorded by micro- or macro-electrodes, as developed by Bertrand (Bertrand, Jasper, Wong, Matthews, 1968). Beckman DC electrodes, arranged after Kris (Kris 1960), were used to record the electro-oculogram (EOG). Low impedance electrodes were connected directly to a Schwarzer EEG machine while high impedance electrodes were first connected to a Picometric amplifier. The longest AC time constant, 3 sec, was used to record EOGs. All recordings were monopolar and the surface area of each thalamic electrode was measured. The indifferent point was provided by biaural leads connected by a 20K Ω resistor bridge or by a bridged neck-chest lead; the stereotaxic frame served as ground. All records were visually analyzed usually a blind procedure wherein each channel was individually examined, the position of a noteworthy event marked and the total record subsequently re-examined.

Target points for deep recording sites were reconstructed from X-ray photographs and micrometer readings of electrode extension and the reconstructions were matched to sections in the atlas of Schaltenbrand and Bailey (Schaltenbrand, Bailey, 1959). Confirmation of electrode placement (via lesion location) was obtained in several patients who came to postmortem examination. Twenty-eight points were recorded from in the nucleus pulvinaris; fourteen in the pulvinaris orolateralis, eight in the pulvinaris oroventralis, and six in the pulvinaris medialis.

Constant current stimuli—6 or 60 pulses per sec (pps), 1 msec pulse width, 1–10 sec train duration, electrode tip negative—were generated by a Grass S4 stimulator in conjunction with the Picometric amplifier. Current density never exceeded 750 $\mu$A/cm$^2$/pulse, usually being less than 500 $\mu$A/cm$^2$/pulse; the density needed for larger electrodes was naturally less (Libet, Alberts, Wright, Delattre, Levin, Feinstein, 1964). No gross movements, pain or other sensations or speech alterations were observed or reported at these current densities.

Subjects were required to fixate, alternate among fixation points, or follow a pendulum at 2.7 m or 32 cm distance; subjects also read material at 32 cm distance. Material presented at 2.7 m subtended a visual angle of 10° 30', that at 32 cm, 28°, reading material, 14°. All material was illuminated by a multibeam surgical lamp.

## RESULTS

Pulvinar and cortical alpha rhythms and oculomotor activity are examined under five conditions: 1) rest, eyes closed; 2) eye closure; 3) fixation-holding, smooth pursuit (pendulum following); 4) saccadic eye movements; 5) pulvinar stimulation. For these data comparison is made between the electrical activity at one pulvinar locus and that at many cortical loci, more cortical loci than would satisfy the known anatomical projections of the pulvinar; it is not possible in these experiments to record from directly connected cortical and pulvinar loci. The data are equivalent whether a macro- or a micro-electrode is used in recording from deep structures. In this report we shall follow, with slight modification, the terminology laid down by Anderson *et al.* (Andersen, Andersson, Lømo, 1967) for cortical and thalamic spindle waves.

### 1. Rest

Although pulvinar and cortical alpha rhythms frequently appear concurrently (compound cortico-thalamic alpha) (about 73 percent of occurrences) alpha rhythm may appear in either structure (local alpha) without appearing in the other.

Even when they appear concurrently the two alpha rhythms may differ in the time of start and stop of the activity, the intra-alpha wave frequency and amplitude as well as in the frequency of appearance and inter-alpha period (Fig. 1). These differences are maintained independent of the amount of cortical alpha activity demonstrated by a given patient. If the thalamic alpha rhythm is unaccompanied by cortical alpha during a 3 sec period preceding and succeeding it we are terming this event "isolated thalamic alpha." Isolated thalamic alpha is associated with 3 percent of pulvinar alpha occurrences. In a few cases a good relationship exists in terms of intra-alpha wave frequency (a well correlated phase relationship) between the pulvinar and the frontal cortex. (An anatomical projection from the frontal eye field to the medial pulvinar

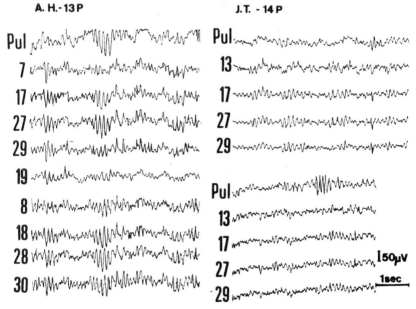

Figure 5–1. Three examples of the variable relationships between alpha rhythm appearance and form in the pulvinar and at various scalp positions. Recording points not shown include 6 and 20; they showed no alpha pattern. Left (A.H.-13P) alpha rhythm is prominent both in the depth and on the surface. Right (J.T.-14P) above, alpha is largely restricted to the surface and below it is most prominent in the pulvinar. Pulvinar recording site for A.H.-13P and J.T.-14P, pulvinaris orolateralis.

has been demonstrated (Trachtenberg, Akert, unpublished data).

## 2. Eye closure.

Eye closure, particularly after strenuous visuo-motor activity is a potent generator of cortical alpha rhythm; 96 percent of eye closures are followed by alpha appearance. Eye closure frequently (81 percent of occurrences) evokes a pulvinar alpha rhythm; of these 2 percent are isolated thalamic alpha. Obviously then, in almost no case does a pulvinar alpha appear without some cortical alpha being present in the record. This does not mean that compound corticothalamic alpha is the rule as the alpha onset time and order are particularly variable (Fig. 2). When compound cortico-thalamic alpha is seen the

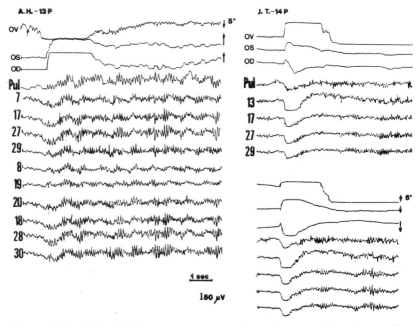

Figure 5–2. Alpha rhythm generation in the pulvinar and on the surface induced by eye closure. Left (A.H.-13P), alpha onset is nearly simultaneous in the pulvinar and scalp leads 27 and 29. Right (J.T.-14P) above, alpha appears first at the surface, below, alpha is first seen in the pulvinar. OV-vertical EOG recording, OS-horizontal EOG from the left eye, OD-horizontal EOG from the right eye. Arrows point to upwards or rightwards eye movements. Pulvinar recording sites as in Fig. 1.

phase relationships of individual waves tend to become variable with time.

### 3. Fixation-holding

A burst of alpha will appear at scalp leads with losses of fixation (as judged from EOG records) either while the subject fixates or during pendulum following (Pollen, Trachtenberg, 1972). Loss of fixation is a moderately potent alpha generator either in the pulvinar or the cortex and the likelihood of a compound cortico-thalamic alpha wave is slight (Fig. 3). An

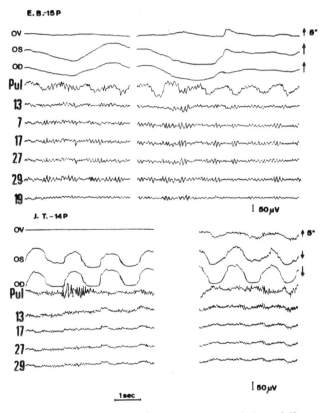

Figure 5–3. Alpha bursting during lapses in pendulum following; pendulum at 2.7 m distance. Above (E.G.-15P), alpha appears in both pulvinar and at the surface usually starting at the surface. Below (J.T.-14P) prominent alpha bursting is restricted to the pulvinar. Pulvinar recording sites, E.B.-15P, pulvinaris orolateralis, J.T.-14P as in Fig. 1.

alpha rhythm can be seen in cortical and pulvinar records 67 percent of the times while it is apparent in the cortical records about 85 percent of the times. Isolated thalamic alpha occupies 4 percent of pulvinar alpha occurrences. As with eye closure, alpha may have its earliest onset in the scalp records, in the pulvinar, or it may appear simultaneously at both loci. However, as with eye closure, the pulvinar alpha rhythm is generally far more prominent in terms of its amplitude and burst-like appearance than is the cortical alpha, and at times the pulvinar alpha exceeds 12 cps. All isolated thalamic alpha is of this burst-like appearance. During pulvinar bursts the patient appears drowsy though he continues to perform his visual task adequately, i.e. he gives the appearance of being an automaton. Although we have seen only eleven such instances, the correlation of behavior and electrophysiology in this situation is one.

### 4. Saccadic movements

While the subject is reading, making good saccadic eye movements, a pulvinar alpha rhythm does not appear and alpha is rarely obvious at the cortex. Alpha is also absent when the patient alters his fixation point, at either 32 cm or 2.7 m, though sporadic alpha appears in the cortex and/or pulvinar after sustained fixation. Particularly at these latter times, along with the presence of pulvinar alpha, the patient would appear bored or drowsy.

### 5. Pulvinar stimulation

Pulvinar stimulation at 6 pps, at a current density of no more than 750 $\mu$A/cm$^2$/pulse, is without effect on eye movements or cortical EEG patterns, save the rare appearance of a cortical EEG slowing (e.g. from 12 to 8 cps). Stimulation at 60 pps, however, alters both the alpha rhythm and oculomotor movements; verbal reports confirm the latter. The latency to either alteration may be 5–8 sec and requires stimuli of several seconds duration indicating that extensive facilitation is required and suggesting the involvement of polysynaptic pathways. Fig. 4A shows cortical alpha generation with pulvinar stimulation. The cortically generated alpha is bila-

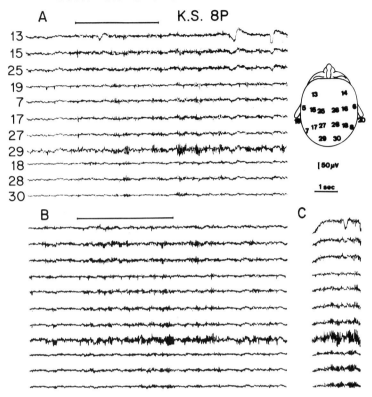

Figure 5–4. Surface alpha generation with pulvinar stimulation. A. Little alpha present before stimulation; clear delayed onset with post-stimulus alpha continuing. B. Alpha enhancement by pulvinar stimulation. Latency of effect reduced as compared with A. Stimuli delivered during the period indicated by black bar. C. Alpha release when pendulum, at 2.7 m, is suddenly stopped. Compare pattern with A and B. Pulvinar stimulation site, pulvinaris orolateralis. Right, schematic drawing illustrating the various recording points used.

teral though weaker and of greater latency contralaterally. If a cortical alpha rhythm is initially present, stimulation will enhance it (Fig. 4B); again this enhancement is bilateral. A comparison of Fig. 4A and B with C indicates the efficacy of this type of stimulation as opposed to natural stimuli. Fig. 4C shows the alpha appearance, eyes open, immediately after sudden cessation of the pendulum to which the subject had been attending. Pulvinar stimulation is a more potent alpha

generator on the ipsilateral side; the alpha amplitude attains
70–80 percent of that seen in response to a natural stimulus.
On the contralateral side the evoked alpha rhythm attains
an amplitude only 40–50 percent of that which appears with
a natural trigger stimulus. Although the subject's eyes remain
open and he is instructed to continue to fixate the pendulum,
the cortical alpha rhythm continues as long as 10 seconds
after cessation of stimulation. With stimuli sufficient to generate a cortical alpha rhythm electrode polarization prevents

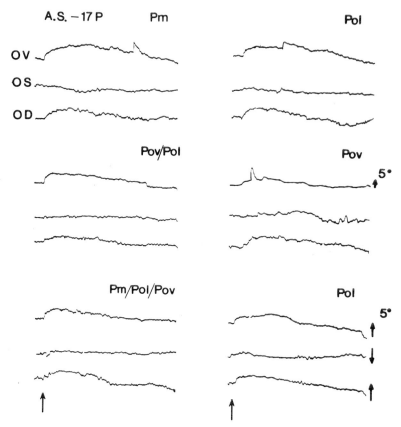

Figure 5–5. EOG alterations induced by pulvinar stimulation at the sites
noted. Traces arranged as a function of alteration in the horizontal position
of the left eye (OS). See text for description. Stimulation in left pulvinar.
Pm=pulvinaris medialis, Pov=pulvinaris oroventralis, Pol=pulvinaris
orolateralis, slash indicates border regions.

a view of the evoked pulvinar activity. When the trace returns, 15–30 sec later, no alteration of activity is noted. An extensive study of thalamic sites yielding cortical alpha rhythm was not undertaken but stimulation of the ventralis anterior, ventralis lateralis or dorsalis medialis at similar current densities does not result in the generation of cortical alpha rhythm.

Some of the time an EEG activation precedes alpha appearance. Then EOG alterations are visable. Fig. 5 shows the EOG alterations induced by pulvinar stimulation (in an anesthetized patient). Stimulation of every locus in the left pulvinar results in an oblique upward-rightward movement of the right eye. The left eye shows a small amplitude horizontal deviation which varies from slightly rightward to leftward. Similar stimulation in an unanesthetized patient, fixating a point 2.7 m distant, is accompanied by a report of sudden diplopia. However, neither alpha generation nor EOG activation follow pulvinar stimulation while the subject is reading.

No EEG or EOG alterations are seen when a similarly anesthetized, control subject is stimulated at any of four sites in the dorsalis medialis thalamus with currents up to 50 percent greater than those used in the pulvinar.

## DISCUSSION

The data show that cortical and pulvinar EEG activities not only can exhibit considerable variability as regards intra-alpha wave frequency, time of start and stop, and inter-alpha period, but that complete independence of appearance (isolated thalamic alpha) can and does occur. Both the variability and the independence are maintained even when a discernable trigger event, e.g. eye closure or fixation loss, is available. Independence is more often seen in the latter case. Two arguments might be raised against the significance of these statements: 1) insufficient number of cortical points are recorded from, and 2) thalamo-cortical point-to-point specificity is so precise that direct cortical recording from that cortical point showing maximal evoked potential amplitude must be employed.

As regards the first, we recorded from as many points as possible including all those representing anatomically related sites (e.g. recording sites 7, 17, 27, 9, 19, 20, 15, 16, 29, 30) available on the closed calvarium, and even the use of a macro-electrode did not improve the relationships. However much they may distort phase and onset time relationships, the global recording methods used are exquisitely sensitive to recording the presence or absence of large amplitude rhythmic activity at any cortical locus. Thus, the percentage (9%) of isolated thalamic alpha bursts indicates a more profound independence of thalamus and cortex under these conditions and between these sites than prevails in the barbiturated state (Andersen, Andersson, 1968). In the barbiturated state there is greater receptivity to rhythmic (spindle) activity in both cortex and thalamus than exists under more natural conditions, consequently the likelihood of seeing compound thalamocortical spindles increases and that of seeing isolated spindles decreases. The likelihood of generating cortical EEG spindle activity by stimulation of any thalamic nucleus also increases. In the nonanesthetized state there is a general correlation between cortical and thalamic rhythmic activity-frontal and parietal cortices show less alpha than occipito-temporal cortices, the thalamic nuclei with which they are connected also show little or no alpha while the pulvinar alone shows prominent alpha rhythm. The dorsalateral thalamus (including pulvinar) is relatively independent of driving from the medial thalamus and may show well developed spindles while the medial and ventrobasal thalamic groups are spindle free (Andersson, Manson, 1971). Also, stimulation of non-pulvinar sites does not generate cortical alpha at anywhere near the currents suitable when stimulating the pulvinar.

The cortices having the most prominent alpha, areas 18, 19 and their surrounding regions receive connections primarily from the pulvinar (Chow, 1950; Cragg, Ainsworth, 1969; Locke, 1960), in addition to their extensive intracortical connections (Kuypers, Szwarcbart, Mishkin, Rosvold, 1965; Pandya, Kuypers, 1969), while area 17 receives exclusively from the lateral geniculate body (Whitlock, Nauta, 1956). It is not unreasonable to assume that each thalamic nucleus acts upon its cortical regions independently of the other. Thus information could be processed in the lateral geniculate body, areas 17, 18 and 19, while the pulvinar, particularly its medial and oral divisions, remains at rest, exhibiting an alpha pattern. (Cowey and Gross, 1970) support the idea of regional independence of function in those cortical visual areas connected to the pulvinar. They suggest that the foveal prestriate regions are concerned with visual attention or perception and the inferotemporal cortex with the associative or mnemonic stage of visual processing. The observation of oral pulvinar alpha burst and automaton-like behavior fits this suggestion well.

When the visuo-motor system becomes locked into a response pattern and no associative visual processing is necessary, the pulvinar zero output modulation may be seen in the cortex as an "idling" pattern—the alpha rhythm. When considerable pulvinar output modulation is present it should be difficult to induce a cortical alpha rhythm. This is in agreement with our inability to induce cortical alpha by pulvinar stimulation while the subject was involved in tasks such as reading which demand high acuity and are accompanied by little cortical alpha (Pollen, Trachtenberg, 1972). If the pulvinar is involved in resolving fine detail, under such circumstances significant oculomotor control should be exercised and pulvinar stimulation should be unable to affect eye position; this is the case when the subject is visually and intellectually active.

Before considering the effects of stimulation in further detail two points require clarification: a) specificity of the site of stimulation and b) the neural elements stimulated. Stimulation of the dorsalis medialis thalamus of a control patient produces neither EEG nor EOG alteration. Likewise stimulation of the ventralis lateralis thalamus in these subjects does not result in alpha rhythm appearance or eye movements, at the parameters used. Also, the use of a microelectrode for stimulation serves to restrict the stimulated region. These observations lead us to conclude that pulvinar structures are responsible for the observed effects.

The pulvinar contains the internal corticotectal tract carrying fibers presumably concerned with ocular fixation and holding. It is very difficult to be sure that pulvinar neurons are being activated as opposed to this fiber system. However, the oral and medial divisions of the pulvinar are free of this fiber system and stimulation of several different regions, having different relationships with traversing fibers, give similar EEG and EOG reactions. It is not possible to decide, from these experiments, which classes of neurons are being activated—those associated with the cortex or those associated with the tectum or with other loci. Crighel* has shown that evoked potentials can be recorded in one pulvinar while stimulating the other in the precollicular cat, in which spreading depression is induced in one cortex. This argues for a diencephalic connection between the two pulvinars. This finding may provide an anatomical basis, in addition to the corpus collowum, for the efficacy of pulvinar induced cortical alpha contralaterally as well as ipsilaterally. What anatomical pathway can account for the contralateral disconjugate eye movements induced by pulvinar stimulation? We propose that pulvinar efferents cross the brain stem in the posterior commissure and then run, with intervening synapses, to the various oculomotor nuclei; activation of cortical or tectal pathways would be expected to result in conjugate deviation.

Alpha rhythm generation is a complex response and as such exhibits different latencies in response to stimulation at different loci and even to the same locus at different times. The latter indicates the varying receptivity, i.e., differing state of cortical neurons, to rhythmic activation and the involvement of polysynaptic pathways. As expected, a priori, pulvinar stimulation results in large amplitude alpha waves ipsilaterally and once set into rhythmic activity the cortex continues for some seconds after cessation of the stimulus. The cortical alpha amplitude attains a large percentage of that appearing in response to natural stimuli indicating the strength of pulvinar influence on cortical activity.

A given stimulus can evoke a cortical alpha rhythm and/or

---

* Personal Communication

an oculomotor movement. Does any relationship exist between these phenomena? While we cannot answer this question definitively at this time, we feel that a relationship does exist: when both alpha and eye movements appear, alpha generation tends to follow an eye movement and eye movements are preceded by EEG activation.

## SUMMARY

Physiological investigations are carried out in the pulvinar of humans at neurosurgical operation.

1. EEG recordings taken from both pulvinar and cortical loci show that EEG dissociation can occur between the cortex and pulvinar such that thalamic alpha can be recorded with little relationship to, and in some cases in the absence of, any rhythmic cortical activity. This phenomenon is observable even in the presence of defined trigger events such as eye closure or fixation loss. The behavioral concomitant of pulvinar alpha bursts is an automoton-like appearance.

2. High frequency, low current density, stimulation of the pulvinar is followed by the generation or enhancement of a cortical alpha rhythm. Response latencies may be 5–8 sec indicating the action of multisynaptic pathways and extensive facilitation. This phenomenon occurs whether the patient's eyes are open or closed. If the eyes are open, considerable voluntary oculomotor control, as in reading, appears to prevent induced alpha generation.

3. Pulvinar stimulation can directly influence oculomotor behavior after similar latency. Pulvinar stimulation can result in disconjugate eye movements with the major effects on the eye contralateral to the site of stimulation. Patients report diplopia at this time. Patterned oculomotor movements prevent these stimulation induced movements.

## References

Albe-Fessard, D., Arfel, G., et Guiot, G., Derome, P., Hertzog, E., Vourc, H.G., Brown, N.H., Aleonard, P., DeLaherran, J., and Trigo, J.C.: Electrophysiological studies of some deep cerebral structures in man. *J. Neurol. Sci.* 3:37–51, 1966.

Andersen, P., and Andersson, S.A.: *Physiological Basis of the Alpha Rhythm*. N.Y., Appleton-Century-Crofts, pp. 235, 1968.

Andersen, P., Andersson, S.A. and Lømo, T.: Nature of thalamocortical relations during spontaneous barbiturate spindle activity. *J. Physiol. (Lond.) 192:*283–307, 1967.

Andersson, S.A., Holmgren, E. and Manson, J.R.: Synchronization and desynchronization in the thalamus of the unanesthetized decorticate cat. *Electroenceph. clin. Neurophysiol. 31:*335–346, 1971.

Andersson, S.A., Holmgren, E. and Manson, J.R.: Localized thalamic rhythmicity induced by spinal and cortical lesions. *Electroenceph. clin. Neurophysiol. 31:*347–363, 1971.

Andersson, S.A. and Manson, J.R.: Rhythmic activity in the thalamus of the unanesthetized decorticate cat. *Electroenceph. clin. Neurophysiol. 31:*21–34, 1971.

Bertrand, G., Jasper, H., Wong, A., and Mathews, G.: Microelectrode recording during stereotactic surgery. *Clin. Neurosurg. 16:*328–355, 1968.

Campos-Ortega, J.A., Hayhow, W.R. and Cluver, P.F. deV. A note on the problem of retinal projections to the inferior pulvinar nucleus of primates. *Brain Res. 22:*126–130, 1970.

Chow, K.L.: A retrograde cell degeneration study of the cortical projection field of the pulvinar in the monkey. *J. Comp. Neur. 92:*313–340, 1950.

Cooper, I.S., Waltz, J.M., Amin, I. and Fujita, S.: Pulvinectomy: A preliminary report, *J. Am. Ger. Soc. 19:*553–554, 1971.

Cowey, A. and Gross, C.G.: Effects of foveal prestriate and inferotemporal lesions on visual discrimination by the rhesus monkey. *Exp. Brain Res. 11:*128–144, 1970.

Cragg, B.G. and Ainsworth, A.: The topography of the afferent projections in the circumstriate visual cortex of the monkey studied by the Nauta method. *Vision Res. 9:*733–747, 1969.

Kris, C.: Vision: *Electro-oculography*. In: O. Glaser (Ed.) *Medical Physics*, Chicago, Year Book Publishers, Vol III, pp. 692-700, 1960.

Kuypers, H.G.J.M., Szwarcbart, M.K., Mishkin, M. and Rosvold, H.E.: Occipito-temporal connections in the rhesus monkey. *J. Comp. Neur. 85:*223–305, 1965.

Libet B., Alberts, W.W., Wright, Jr., E.W., DeLattre, L.D., Levin, G., and Feinstein, B.: Production of threshold levels of conscious sensation by electrical stimulation of human somato-sensory cortex. *J. Neurophysiol. 27:*546–578, 1964.

Locke, S.: The projection of the medial pulvinar of the macaque. *J. Comp. Neur. 115:*155–170, 1960.

Mulholland, T.B.: The concept of attention and the electroencephalographic alpha rhythm. In: Evans, C.R. and Mulholland, T.B. (Eds.), *Attention in Neurophysiology*. N.Y., Appleton-Century-Crofts, pp. 100–127, 1969.

Pandya, D.N. and Kuypers, H.G.J.M.: Cortico-cortical connections in the rhesus monkey. *Brain. Res. 13:*13–36, 1969.

Pollen, D.A., and Trachtenberg, M.C.: Some problems of occipital alpha block in man. *Brain Res. 41*:303–314, 1972.

Rakic, P. and Sidman, R.L.: Telencephalic origin of pulvinar neurons in fetal human brain. Z. *Anat. EntwGesch. 129*:53–82, 1969.

Richardson, D.E. and Zorub, D.S.: Sensory function of the pulvinar. *Confin. neurol. 32*:165–173, 1970.

Schaltenbrand, G., and Bailey, P.: *Introduction to stereotaxis with an atlas of the human brain.* Stuttgart, Georg Thieme Verlag, 1959.

Siegfried, J.: Thalamic surgery in the treatment of pain. *Confin. neurol.* (in press.)

Spatz, W.B., Tigges, J. and Tigges, M.: Subcortical projections, cortical associations, and some intrinsic interlaminar connections of the striate cortex in the squirrel monkey (*Samiri*) *J. Comp. Neur. 140*:155–174, 1970.

Trachtenberg, M.C., and Akert, K.: Projections of the frontal cortex especially the frontal eye fields in the macaque brain. Unpublished data.

Whitlock, D.G., and Nauta, W.J.: Subcortical projections from the temporal neocortex in Macacca mulatta. *J. Comp. Neur. 106*:183–212, 1956.

Wilson, M.E. and Cragg, B.G.: Projections from the lateral geniculate nucleus in the cat and monkey. *J. Anat. (Lond) 101*:677–692, 1967.

Yoshii, N., Adachi, K., Kudo, T., Shimizu, S., Nishioka, S., and Nakahama, H.: Further studies on the stereotaxis thalamotomy for pain relief. *Tohoku J. Exp. Med. 102*:225–232, 1970.

## DISCUSSION

**Dr. Frigyesi:** When the subjects were not solving problems of blindfold chess, there was no blocking of the alpha rhythm. You implied that when information processing is going on, the alpha rhythm is depressed and conversely, when alpha rhythm is present information processing does not take place in the central nervous system. One gets the impression that this generalization goes beyond what is permissible from these data.

**Dr. Trachtenberg:** Perhaps we have overstated the case. What we mean to put forth is that attention directed towards fine detail is associated with alpha block in the situation of blindfold chess playing. As I showed, as the subject became more acclimated to the task, the alpha became more prominent. Now, if a deliberate incorrect move was made by the subject's opponent, or a move that would not be expected in terms of predictability of chess games, then the subject would show a clear sudden block of the alpha rhythm indicat-

ing that he now had to exercise increased mental effort in
order to deal with this contingency (Pollen and Trachtenberg,
1972). I used the term "information processing" in a restricted
sense, one which is particularly related to problem solving
activity.

**Dr. Frigyesi:** It is known that when a subject attends a
task reticular activation takes place which is associated with
suppression of activity arising in the medial thalamic nuclei
which are responsible for the generation of low frequency
high amplitude waves in the motor cortex. Another question
relates to the lack of correlation between the 6/sec waves
in the pulvinar and cortex. This may be so, but do you not
think it is difficult to state this from the data you presented?
Earlier in the day, I showed intracellular recordings from
pulvinar neurons. The triggered EPSP-IPSP sequences
exhibited moderate degrees of correlation with the triggered
neocortical negativities.

**Dr. Trachtenberg:** Our data detail two phenomena: one,
the correlation of block of the alpha rhythm and behavior
(Pollen and Trachtenberg, 1972) and, two, the correlation of
cortical (occipital) and pulvinar alpha rhythms. We do not
discuss the underlying mechanism. The original support for
this contention comes not from our work, as you know, but
from the work of Andersson & Lømo (1967) among others,
suggesting that there is a point to point relationship between
the thalamus and the cortex; not only the intralaminar
thalamus, but the so-called sensory nuclei, indeed all specific
nuclei, serve to drive the respective cortical projection sites.
Therefore, if one is stimulating in the caudate, as was shown,
one might expect a very poor correlation between activity
in the motor cortex and pulvinar, since there are no known
anatomic connections between these two structures.

I next wish to draw attention to your use of the word
"attending" which seems to me to be equivalent to the word
"cognizant" whereas we wish to indicate that when a subject
is "paying attention", he is focusing on the details of the problem and is capable of making subtle differentiations. In the
latter condition the alpha is blocked, during other cognitive
behavior, it is present. The problem difficulty necessary to

block the alpha rhythm differs for each person and for any person at different times.

**Dr. Frigyesi:** Sven Andersson recently published some views deviant to those he had published with Per Andersen.

**Dr. Trachtenberg:** Subsequent reading of these articles indicates that Andersson and his colleagues (Andersson and Mason, 1971, Anderson *et al.* 1971, a,b) make the following points relevant to this discussion:

1. Whereas spindle activity in the ventro-basal thalamic nuclei is dependent upon or gated by the medial thalamic nuclei, the spindle activity in the dorso-lateral nuclei (including pulvinar) is rather independent of other thalamic rhythms.

2. The cell population responsible for spindle generation varies with time.

3. There are multiple rhythmic generators in the thalamus imposing rhythmic activity on the cortex.

4. "That the rhythmic activity in a cortical projection area is largely determined by the discharge pattern of thalmo-cortical fibres arising from the corresponding specific thalamic nuclei . . . "

5. With the loss of a specific input (as by spinal cord section) rhythmic activity increases in thalamic and topographically related cortical loci, loci which receive this specific input.

6. Thalamic spindle activity is not dependent on either the cortex or the mesencephalic reticular formation therefore, all of the appropriate circuits for spindle generation are intrinsic to the thalamus.

**Dr. Frigyesi:** Another point I wish to remind you of: In your data you showed that pulvinar stimulation triggers, under certain conditions, relatively high frequency response, that you have shown operating in the cortex. How can you reconcile this statement with the work that was presented by Dr. Crighel earlier today, in which he indicated that the pulvinar stimulation at no matter what frequency he used, fails to effect the electro-cortical tracings?

**Dr. Trachtenberg:** I think there is very little further that can be said, reconciling Dr. Crighel's data with ours, save perhaps for the fact that we are working with humans and

Dr. Crighel has been working with cats. As for your first comment, I don't argue that rhythmic activity may be roving from one place in the thalamus to another, likewise it roves from one place in the cortex to another. The point we are stressing, as put forth by Andersen and his colleagues, is that at any given point in time there is a relationship between cortical and thalamic activity, in two points which are anatomically connected. Similarly Pollen (personal communication) has repeatedly emphasized the rigorous topographical relationship existing between thalamic and cortical loci as judged by evoked potential amplitude or efficacy in generating spindle or spike and wave potentials.

**Dr. Gilman:** I would like to throw some fuel on the fire if I may. I do believe that some of the work that Dr. Frigyesi has alluded to, namely Dr. Andersen's thesis, has been essentially refuted and partially retracted. I think, though, that Dr. Trachtenberg's observations are extremely interesting and of great importance. I would cite one of his observations alone as being of great significance and this is the observation that pulvinar stimulation produced ocular movements. One of the current views in neuro-opthalmology is that there are two separable types of eye movements. One is saccadic eye movements and the second is pursuit eye movements. Hoyt, Daroff and their colleagues have developed reasonably convincing evidence to indicate that saccadic eye movements are driven from the frontal lobe and pursuit eye movements, which are smooth movements, are driven from occipital lobe. The findings that you demonstrated are highly suggestive to me of the possibility that you are stimulating the tracking motion of the eyes instead of saccadic eye movements and it seems possible that your pulvinar stimulation, by way of an occipital cortical route, is driving the smooth pursuit-type movement. I believe this idea bears further investigation. Incidentally, contrary to our common conception that most central nervous system control affects the contralateral side of the body, Hoyt has put forth the hypothesis that the ipsilateral occipital cortex has an ipsilateral effect on eye movements.

**Dr. Trachtenberg:** I wish to point out that our electrode was in the medial or oral parts of the pulvinar, the same places which Dr. Siqueira has shown do not have through-going fibers from the cortico-tectal and cortico-tegmental tracts. In view of the low current intensities we were using, we should be able to rule out any spurious stimulation of these fiber tracts. This allows me to suggest more strongly that we are really affecting the cortex, and then, perhaps, indirectly, those fiber tracts.

**Question from floor:** Were these eye movements individual? In other words they weren't conjugated? Is that correct?

**Dr. Trachtenberg:** That's correct.

**Question from floor:** How do you explain that?

**Dr. Trachtenberg:** At present we can only hypothecate.

**Question from floor:** How did you get these conjugate eye movements? You either have to be in the nucleus or below, in the pathways connecting the two individual nuclei.

**Dr. Trachtenberg:** This finding is obviously difficult to explain. On the one hand, I note that in addition to pulvinar-cortical fibers, and cortical-pulvinar fibers there are tecto-pulvinar and cortico-tectal fibers, any of which may be stimulated in this situation, and to what degree each system is stimulated I cannot say. On the other, in view of Dr. Crighel's work, we suggest that the pulvinar provides a crossed descending output to the oculomotor nuclei via the posterior commissure.

**Dr. Crighel:** I want to say that the differences between our results after the tetanization of the pulvinar and yours are not only because of the differences in species but also because of your very long lasting stimulation. We stimulated with 100/sec only with 50 ms duration of the stimulating burst and not longer than 300 ms. Your stimulating burst lasted 1–10 sec.

**Dr. Trachtenberg:** That's right.

# CHAPTER 6

# PSYCHOLOGICAL FUNCTIONS FOLLOWING PULVINECTOMY IN MAN

M. Riklan, Ph.D., D. Weissman, M.A. and
I.S. Cooper, M.D., Ph.D.

THERE NOW EXISTS a fairly extensive body of literature with respect to the psychological effects of surgically placed lesions in various thalamic nuclei in man. In addition, some data are also available concerning behavioral effects of stimulation to such nuclei. Concerning the psychological consequences of lesions placed in the ventrolateral (VL) nucleus in the parkinsonian, a review of findings was recently undertaken by Riklan and Levita (1969). They noted, generally, that the parkinsonian's preoperative level of behavioral and cerebral integration was closely related to the degree of psychological alteration observed both immediately postoperatively and in longer range postoperative assessment. During the period immediately following VL surgery, a time ranging from 5 to 21 days after surgery, losses in some integrative functions were associated with unilateral lesions. Such deficits were not necessarily related to a single anatomic structure but seemed rather to reflect a general physiological disruption of neural functions. In the follow-up situation, 6 months or more after surgery, mean psychological test scores had returned to their preoperative level. These findings were interpreted as a lack of specific behavioral effects associated with unilateral subcortical lesions probably related to cerebral plasticity and/or equipotentiality. It was suggested that small lesions placed within larger functional systems permit the

138

remaining tissues to undertake the functions involved. Finally, apparent lack of longer range effects might also reflect test insensitivity to subtle "nonspecific" behavioral alterations.

Immediate postoperative and longer range observations of patients subjected to bilateral thalamic surgery have suggested a decrease in "nonspecific activation, energy, or drive" (Riklan, Levita, and Coper, 1966). Such bilateral surgery ordinarily involves two consecutive operations, with second surgery usually following unilateral operation by a period of at least 6 months. Alterations in language and speech have also been observed in conjunction with both unilateral and bilateral thalamic surgery. Changes in verbal functions tend to be more pronounced with left than with right hemisphere lesions, though no gross qualitative differences could be reported as a function of lesion laterality. Alterations in speech, which may occasionally occur after unilateral surgical intervention, tend to be more frequently associated with bilateral operations regardless of the cerebral hemisphere involved in the second operation. In general, follow-up psychological tests of verbal functions have not consistently shown changes associated with unilateral or bilateral subcortical lesions. Furthermore, within a zone encompassing the ventrolateral area of the thalamus, variations in size or site of surgical lesions were not consistently related to postoperative changes in psychological functions. To the extent that any particular psychological functions can be associated with the ventrolateral thalamus, they may involve primarily a contribution of activation, arousal, or attention to the neural factors underlying integrated behavior. A relatively "unrefined" stage of data processing and elaboration has been associated with these structures and systems and might provide some justification for this tentative suggestion.

Not all investigators have agreed that discrete lesions in the area of the thalamus fail to result in long range behavioral changes in the parkinsonian. For example, Meier and Story (1967) administered the Porteus Maze preoperatively and 8 months postoperatively to a series of patients in whom subthalamic lesions were placed in the region of the fields of forel. They found a selective impairment in Maze performance, only after right subthalamotomy, in the absence of alterations in global intelligence. Jurko and Andy (1964) reported that "diencephalotomy" in parkinsonians resulted in long range impairment in a test involving concept formation, from a standard IQ test, up to 2 years postoperatively. However, neither of these reports dealt exclusively with ventrolateral thalamic lesions. In contrast, Perret and Siegfried (1969) tested 18 parkinsonians before and after unilateral ventrolateral thalamotomy. These authors reported that neither verbal or performance I.Q. scores were appreciably affected by such surgery. However, in three learning and memory tests, thalamotomy was followed by a longer range decrement in performance.

Recently some data have become available concerning pulvinar stimulation and lesions in man. The pulvinar is the largest thalamic nucleus in man, and along with the dorsomedial nucleus, has undergone the greatest phyletic expansion over the mammalian series. The principal thalamic connections of the pulvinar are with the medial and lateral geniculate bodies, lateral and central nuclear groups, and the dorsomedial nucleus (Walker, 1938, 1966; LeGros Clark and Northfield, 1937). Papez (1939) has reviewed the evidence for connections with amygdala and piriform cortex. In addition, there are major reciprocal connections with the parietal cortex. The medial nucleus of the pulvinar projects mainly to the posterior parietal region, and lateral nucleus to posterior temporal lobe (Simpson, 1952; Truex and Carpenter, 1969). Van Buren and Borke (1969) have suggested, on the basis of degeneration studies in a few aphasic cases, that the anterior superior pulvinar is in relation to the temporoparietal speech area. In cats, evoked responses in the pulvinar were noted following cutaneous stimulation (Richardson & Zorub, 1969). Kreindler, Crighel, and Marinchescu (1968) demonstrated recently that, in cats, visual, auditory and somatic afferents converge in the same neuronal pools in the pulvinar-lateralis posterior complex (PUL-LP). Such pools were found, also, to have projections to homolateral and contralateral neocortical association areas. These authors suggested that the PUL-LP complex is part of a large integrating system, including the associative nuclei of the thalamus, the neocortex (both associative and primary areas), and the thalamic nuclei of diffuse projection necessary to the modulation and control of the afferent systems.

Following lesions or stimulation of the pulvinar in man some behavioral alterations have been observed. For example, Kudo, Yoshii, Shimizu, Aikawa and Nishioka (1968) placed pulvinar lesions in 17 patients suffering from chronic pain. Included were 9 bilateral operations, 4 left hemisphere, and 2 right hemisphere operations. In addition, 2 other patients had bilateral operations with surgery several months apart. These investigators reported that in 5 patients no behavioral changes were noted. However, 8 patients were "easily moved to tears" for several days postoperatively, 2 patients were cheerful, one excitable, and one childish. No long term emotional or evidently any other behavioral changes were noted. Richardson (1967) placed unilateral and bilateral lesions in thalamic nuclei including centrum medianum, posterior centrum medianum, and anterior pulvinar in 38 patients with intractable pain, reporting no instance of gross mental, emotional or behavioral change.

Cooper (1971, 1972) recently described the use of cryopulvinectomy for the alleviation of intractable pain, spasticity, and other hypertonic disorders. Preliminary studies of language and cognition following such surgical lesions (Brown, Riklan, Waltz, Jackson, and Cooper, 1971) indicated that individuals with normal preoperative language and cognition can undergo unilateral right or left pulvinectomy without major alteration during the immediate postoperative period. However, individuals with acquired preoperative deficits in language or signs of "organicity" on psychological tests tended to show further regression following unilateral pulvinectomy. Behavioral changes have been mild and of a questionable nature. Moreover, three patients with bilateral lesions placed in the pulvinar demonstrated no gross evidence of language or cognitive impairment according to a recent study of Brown, Riklan, and Cooper (1972). In two of these patients immediate postoperative I.Q. testing showed a slight decrement. One patient who demonstrated a longer term decrement in cognitive function was under heavy medication for dystonia, and it is quite likely that this contributed to the continuing decline in performance. Such results confirmed the preliminary findings that no marked untoward language, cognitive, or behavioral alterations appear to result from either unilateral or bilateral pulvinar lesions placed in patients whose preoperative mental function is adequately integrated and where no apparent preoperative deficits (e.g., signs of "organicity") are present.

Ojemann and his co-workers (1968, 1971a,b) described the effects of ventrolateral (VL) and pulvinar (Pul) stimulations in man. Stimulation in the left Pul and left and right deep parietal white substance resulted in anomia (1968). In like manner, stimulation of the left VL thalamus resulted in anomia and perseveration during object naming, as well as alterations in short-term verbal memory (1971a,b). In this latter respect, left VL stimulation only during the recall of an object name resulted in a significant increase in errors of short term recall of verbal material. However, when left VL stimulation was undertaken both during presentation of the stimulus and recall, a significant reduction in recall errors was noted, in contrast to stimulation during recall only. For right VL stimulation, no changes in recall were noted nor was anomia produced. It is important to note here that the behavioral effects of thalamic stimulation cannot be considered comparable to the effects of lesion placement, particularly since in most instances post-lesion testing is undertaken days or months following surgery and whereas stimulation observations are made only during the time of actual stimulation and immediately before or after. Furthermore, the physiological alterations resulting from stimulation and lesion placement may also be presumed to be of a different nature.

It is the purpose of the present study to present psychological data on the effects of pulvinar lesions placed in humans, to relate them to previous findings concerning other thalamic lesions in humans, and to consider conepts of the role of the pulvinar and other thalamic nuclei in behavior.

## POPULATION AND PROCEDURE

The population consisted of 32 consecutively tested patients who underwent VL thalamic or pulvinar surgery. Data concerning surgical technique and pathological confirmation of lesion placement have been presented elsewhere (Cooper, Amin, *et al.*,1972) and will not be repeated here. The therapeutic goals of ventrolateral thalamic and pulvinar surgery have also been detailed elsewhere (Cooper, 1961; Cooper, 1969; Cooper *et al.*, 1971; Cooper *et al.*, 1972). Table 1 presents data on age, sex, handedness, diagnosis, and lesion side and site for the patients included in this study.

The sample includes both children and adults whose ages ranged from 11 to 64 years. The younger group, those generally below 25 years of age, includes primarily patients with dystonia musculorum deformans or cerebral palsy, and one patient with epilepsy. Among the older group are included patients with a variety of diagnostic entities, among which are included hemiplegia (stroke syndrome), torticollis, concussion, intention tremor, intractable pain, and parkinsonism. This heterogeneity of diagnostic classification permits for a differential analysis of the psychological test data on the basis of various diagnostic categories. There were 17 males and 15 females. Twenty-two patients were right-handed, 8 were left-handed, and 2 were ambidexterous. Twenty patients underwent left thalamic surgery and 12 underwent right-sided surgery. Of the total group, 16 patients had lesions placed in the pulvinar only (usually 2 lesions, 1 lateral and 1 medial), 9 patients had lesions placed in the VL (or VL and ventroposterolateral) thalamus, and 4 had lesions placed both in the VL nucleus and pulvinar. Three patients had other combinations of lesions. In all instances specific lesion placement was determined by therapeutic needs. The different lesion placements provided the basis in the psychological studies

TABLE 1

THE POPULATION

AGE, SEX, HANDEDNESS, DIAGNOSIS, LESION SIDE AND SITE

| Patient No. | Age | Sex | Handedness | Diagnosis° | Lesion Side | Site°° |
|---|---|---|---|---|---|---|
| 1 | 51 | M | R | Concussion, R. Hemipar. | L | PUL |
| 2 | 11 | F | R | DMD | L | PUL |
| 3 | 33 | M | R | C.P. | L | PUL |
| 4 | 45 | M | L | Torticollis | L | PUL |
| 5 | 41 | F | R | C.P. | R | PUL |
| 6 | 21 | M | R | Epilepsy | R | PUL |
| 7 | 13 | F | Ambidex. | DMD | L | PUL |
| 8 | 10 | F | R | DMD | L | PUL |
| 9 | 29 | M | R | C.P. | R | PUL |
| 10 | 34 | M | R | Athetosis | R | PUL |
| 11 | 15 | M | R | C.P. | R | PUL |
| 12 | 56 | F | R | Cancer | L | PUL |
| 13 | 50 | M | L | R. Spas. Hemi. | L | PUL |
| 14 | 30 | M | L | C.P. | L | PUL |
| 15 | 38 | F | R | C.P. w. Tortic. | R | PUL |
| 16 | 64 | F | R | Intract. Pain | R | PUL |
| 17 | 13 | F | R | DMD | R | L.P. |
| 18 | 52 | F | R | CVA | L | LP & PUL |
| 19 | 24 | F | L | C.P. | L | LP & PUL |
| 20 | 22 | F | R | DMD | L | VL |
| 21 | 13 | F | R | DMD | R | VL |
| 22 | 15 | M | L | Post CVA–L. Hemi. | R | VL |
| 23 | 13 | F | R | DMD | R | VL |
| 24 | 16 | M | R | DMD | L | VL |
| 25 | 60 | M | R | Int. Tremor | L | VL & VPL |
| 26 | 19 | F | Ambidex. | DMD | L | VL & VPL |
| 27 | 44 | M | R | P.D. | L | VL |
| 28 | 16 | M | L | DMD | L | VL |
| 29 | 26 | M | L | C.P. | L | VL & PUL |
| 30 | 20 | M | L | C.P. | L | VL & PUL |
| 31 | 14 | F | R | DMD | L | VL & PUL |
| 32 | 16 | M | R | C.P. | R | VL & PUL |

° DMD–Dystonia Musculorum Deformans  
CP–Cerebral Palsy  
CVA–Cerebrovascular Accident  
P.D.–Parkinson's Disease

°° PUL–Pulvinar  
LP–Lateral Posterior nuc.  
VL–Ventrolateral nuc.  
VPL–Ventroposterolateral nuc.

for methodological control and for comparisons of effect of lesions of different sites and sides.

Of the 32 patients who underwent unilateral thalamic surgery, 3 of these eventually underwent second side thalamic surgery and were evaluated before and after second operations. Because of the small number of patients involved in bilateral operations, statistical analysis will not be undertaken. Rather, individual case reports will be presented and considered.

## PROCEDURE

Routinely patients underwent baseline psychological evaluation between one and three days prior to surgery. Immediate postoperative testing was performed a mean of 8 days following surgery, with the vast majority of patients being tested between 5 and 10 days postoperatively. Long range testing was administered when patients returned for neurological follow-up examinations, a mean of 5 months following surgery, with a range of 3.5 to 6 months. Pre and postoperative data were available for all 32 patients under consideration, while long range follow-up data were available for 12 patients.

For purposes of psychological evaluation, it was decided to assess a variety of "integrative" functions, as a preliminary assessment of a possible behavioral sequela of pulvinar lesions. Consequently, a battery of standardized and objective psychological tests were selected which might provide reliable data concerning certain cognitive, perceptual, perceptual-motor, and memory functions. The tests selected were as follows:

### 1. Wechsler Adult Intelligence Scale (WAIS)

This is perhaps the most frequently utilized individual test of intellectual functions. The test provides a variety of subscores designed to assess such cognitive and perceptual areas as general information, comprehension, concept formation, arithmetical ability, perceptual alertness, attention and concentration, spatial functions, perceptual integration, and perceptual-motor performance. Verbal and nonverbal scores can be ascertained on various functions.

### 2. Wechsler Memory Scale Form I

This test is designed to assess memory functions both recent and remote. Subsections include areas concerned wih personal and current information, orientation, verbal and perceptual memory, and the ability to learn new associations.

### 3. Bender Visual-Motor Gestalt Test

This test, which consists of 9 designs which the subject is required to copy while viewing them, is designed to assess aspects of visual perception, motor performance, and visual-motor integration.

With respect to research design, it was decided to administer the same test pre-and postoperatively, since the design of the study permitted for adequate control through comparisons and contrasts of patients having different lesion sites and sides. In addition to test data derived from the standardized tests just noted, other relevant personal and neurological data were available for each patient. Moreover, daily nurses' and doctors' notes were available for the assessment of postoperative aspects of the patient's behavior of interest. Such observations will be noted at relevant times during the data presentation and discussion, particularly for the 3 patients who eventually underwent bilateral pulvinar surgery.

### RESULTS

The presentation of the results will focus initially upon statistical analysis of group scores, with primary emphasis on comparisons of pre to postoperative data for the different lesion sites and sides. In this respect, Figure 1 shows the pre- and immediate postoperative mean scaled subtest scores for the Wechsler Adult Intelligence Scale for 14 patients undergoing pulvinar surgery. Abbreviations used in Figures 1, 2, 3 and 4 are as follows:

| | |
|---|---|
| I = Information | DSym = Digit Symbol |
| C = Comprehension | PC = Picture Completion |
| A = Arithmetic | BD = Block Design |
| S = Similarities | PA = Picture Arrangement |
| DS = Digit Span | OA = Object Assembly |
| V = Vocabulary | |

Observation of Figure 1 indicates that from pre- to postoperatively most of the subtest mean scaled scores show little change, with a general pattern of cognitive and perceptual

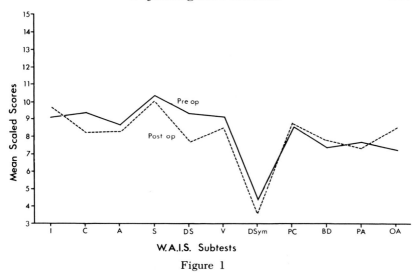

Figure 1

functioning remaining essentially unchanged. In only one subtest, Digit Span, was there a significant reduction in score (p < .05). In this instance, when the left and right hemisphere operates are assessed separately, only scores for the left hemisphere operates were found to be reduced significantly (p < .05). Scores for the Comprehension subtest were decreased somewhat but not significantly, while scores for the Object Assembly subtest were increased somewhat, again not significantly. It may be noted here that the Object Assembly subtest is rather susceptible to practice effects. Figure 2 shows the pre- and postoperative mean subtest scaled scores for the Wechsler Adult Intelligence for 9 patients undergoing ventrolateral thalamic surgery.

As with the pulvinar sample, the pre- to postoperative pattern of subtest scores in the ventrolateral group is essentially unchanged, with only 3 subtest showing alterations. As with the pulvinar lesion, the Digit Span subtest is reduced significantly for the total group (p < .05). However, when left and right hemisphere operates were assessed separately only the left hemisphere group showed a significant decline (p < .05). In addition, the left hemisphere group shows a significant decline in the Similarities and Comprehension subtests (p < .05).

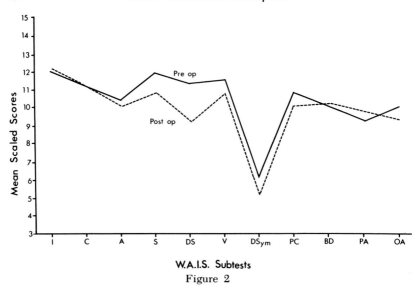

W.A.I.S. Subtests
Figure 2

In essence, with respect to pre-immediate postoperative changes for both the pulvinar and VL groups, the alteration of primary significance is the Digit Span subtest usually considered to represent a measure of attention, concentration, and recent memory. Although scores on this test declined significantly for both lesion groups, the primary contribution to the declines was made by the left hemisphere operates. It may also be noted that when forward and backward Digit Span scores were compared across operative times, no significant differences obtained. In addition, the Similarities and Comprehension subtests declined significantly for the left hemisphere VL patients. It is worthy of note that both of these tests require verbal responses. All other cognitive and perceptual tests remain essentially unchanged from pre- to postoperatively, with the overall pattern of performance also essentially the same. Some data were available concerning longer range follow-up status for both the pulvinar and VL samples. Figure 3 shows the preoperative and long range Wechsler Adult Intelligence Scale subtest scaled scores for 7 patients who underwent pulvinar surgery.

From preoperatively to longer range status only two subtests showed changes of relevance. The Digit Span subtest, which

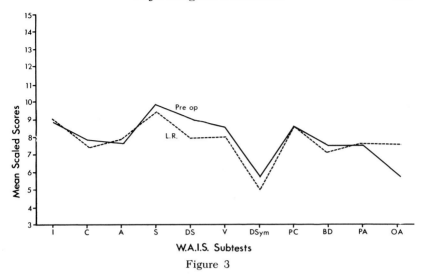

Figure 3

had shown a statistically significant decline during immediate postoperative testing remained somewhat lower than preoperatively, but the decline was not statistically significant. The only significant change was an increase in mean score for the Object Assembly subtest (t = 3.3; p < .02), interpreted here, as previously, as a probable practice or learning effect. Left and right hemisphere operate groups were not assessed separately due to the small numbers involved. Figure 4 shows the preoperative and long range Wechsler Adult Intelligence Scale mean scaled scores for 5 patients who underwent VL surgery.

The pattern of mean long range scores for 5 patients with VL lesions was essentially the same as preoperatively, with slight continuing declines in Comprehension, Picture Completion and Picture Arrangement. These continuing reductions, none of which achieved statistical significance, are due primarily to score decrements of one patient, and should not be interpreted as indicating any group trend.

In addition to statistical analysis of mean scores, some attempt was made to determine which individual patients, both for the pulvinar and VL group, seemed to make the greatest contribution to the score decrements previously described. While such assessment, based as it is upon

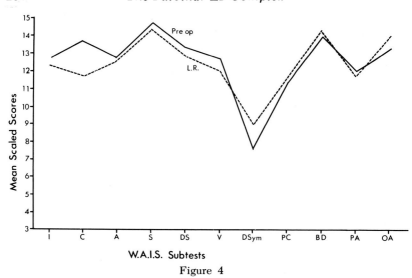

W.A.I.S. Subtests

Figure 4

individual variability, may not be highly reliable, amenable to statistical analysis, or necessarily generalizable to a larger sample, it may provide some clues for further interpretation. Among subjects who showed the greatest immediate post-operative declines in test scores were patients with the following diagnoses: concussion, right hemiplegia, right spastic hemiplegia, torticollis, intention tremor, and cerebral palsy. In 4 out of 5 of these patients pre-existing structural brain damage concomitant with deterioration in integrative, intellectual and perceptual functions were present, as determined by preoperative psychological tests. It was observed also that 3 patients with a diagnosis of dystonia musculorum deformans showed postoperative declines of 10 points or more either in verbal or performance I.Q. score. However, in these 3 instances preoperative performance was well above the sample mean, with full-scale I.Q.'s being 110 or above (mean = 123). It is therefore possible that these patients were manifesting a regression effect, with patients with highest preoperative performance statistically showing a higher tendency for postoperative reductions.

The question of possible lateralized effects of left and right thalamic lesions is of particular relevance in view of the earlier findings of Riklan *et al.* (1960, 1969) and that of Ojemann *et al.* (1968, 1971), concerning a possible differential language or speech function for the left thalamus. Consequently, data were tabulated for both the pulvinar and VL thalamic samples, to show the effects of left and right thalamic surgery on verbal and performance portions of the intelligence test respectively. Table 2 presents the findings.

It is of interest to note that following right hemisphere lesions, for both pulvinar and VL nuclei, no significant pre- to immediate postoperative changes occurred either in verbal or performance tests of cognitive and perceptual functions. However, left hemisphere operates, both pulvinar and VL, showed a differential effect with respect to verbal and performance scores. Specifically, no changes occurred in performance tests, whereas decrements in scores were noted for verbal functions following left hemisphere surgery both for the pulvinar and VL groups. For the VL lesion the pre- to postoperative changes were significant at the $p = .05$ level, based upon a one-tailed test of significance. For pulvinar lesions the decrements showed a similar trend, but did not reach statistical significance. Such data suggest a differential effect both of pulvinar and VL lesions on verbal functions. The implications of this finding will be noted later.

It is of some interest to compare the postoperative changes for the present series of pulvinar and VL lesions with effects of VL and globus pallidus lesions noted in a larger group of parkinsonians to whom a similar test was administered in an earlier study (Riklan *et al.*, 1960). Figure 5 (top portion) shows preoperative, immediate postoperative, and long range postoperative mean scaled scores for 50 parkinsonians tested on the Wechsler Bellevue Scale Form 1.

As indicated on Figure 5, a similar pattern of postoperative changes was noted in the earlier study of parkinsonians undergoing VL thalamus and globus pallidus surgery. Specifically, during the immediate postoperative state a general decline occurred, for the total group, in all of the subtests under consideration. Statistical analysis of the individual subtest scores indicated that only the Digit Span

TABLE 2
PULVINAR AND VENTROLATERAL (OR VL AND VPL) THALAMIC LESIONS
VERBAL–PERFORMANCE I.Q. SCORES–PREOPERATIVE AND IMMEDIATE POSTOPERATIVE
LEFT VS RIGHT THALAMIC SURGERY

| | Left Hemisphere | | | | Right Hemisphere | | | |
| | VIQ | | PIQ | | VIQ | | PIQ | |
| | Pre | Post | Pre | Post | Pre | Post | Pre | Post |
|---|---|---|---|---|---|---|---|---|
| Pulvinar Lesions (N=16) | 99.2 | 89 | 78.1 | 77.5 | 92 | 92.2 | 80.5 | 82.7 |
| Ventrolateral Lesions (N=9) | 114.8 | 106.1 | 102 | 102.2 | 101.3 | 107.6 | 89 | 85.6 |

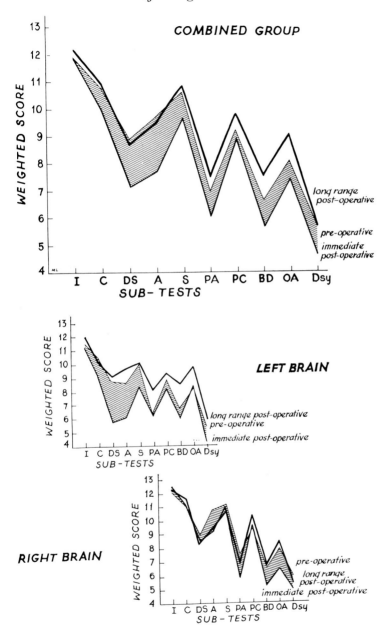

Figure 5

and Digit Symbol subtests were reduced significantly (p = .05). In long range testing all subtest scores had returned to their preoperative level. When patients were separated into left and right hemisphere operates the immediate postoperative and long range scores showed differential alterations, as shown Figure 5 (lower portion).

Figure 5 lower portion indicates that when the left and right hemisphere operates were considered separately postoperatively, the left hemisphere group demonstrated statistically significant greater losses on the Digit Span, Similarities, and Digit Symbol subtests (p = .05). These subtests involve primarily verbal-symbolic responses with the possible exception of the Digit Symbol subtest, which requires perceptual-motor speed and accuracy. For right hemisphere operates the subtest scores showing postoperative decrements were Picture Arrangement, Block Design, and Object Assembly, all requiring perceptual or perceptual-motor performance rather than verbal responses. None of these subtests was reduced to a statistically significant degree. In longer range testing the right brain operates had returned essentially to their preoperative status. The left brain hemisphere operates tend to be higher in performance I.Q. than preoperatively, possibly due to a practice effect.

Perhaps the major difference between the pre-to postoperative test scores for the pulvinar and VL lesion group under consideration here and the VL and globus pallidus group just noted for comparative purposes, is the somewhat greater decrements for the latter sample, immediately postoperatively, in both verbal and performance functions. It is quite possible that this finding is related to the difference in the nature of the two samples. The earlier sample included parkinsonians only whose mean age was 53 with an age range of 31 to 69 years. The current sample, pulvinar and VL cases combined, includes a more heterogeneous group of patients whose mean age is 29 with a range of 11 to 64. Among this group are many younger individuals, particularly dystonics, whose brain and behavior function might be described as more highly integrated than the older patients, and without structural damage. This factor will be considered in further detail.

Some analyses were also undertaken with respect to pre- and postoperative performance on the Bender-Gestalt test by the lesion groups. In this respect it was previously noted that the test was administered while the patient was observing the stimulus. Thus perceptual memory is not a factor. Furthermore, efforts were made, in rating, to discount errors apparently due to the actual motor disabilities manifested by many of the patients. Thus, performance scores are based on the perceptual and perceptual-motor integrative functions tapped by the test rather than possible effects of motor disability. On this basis preoperative Bender-Gestalt scores were rated 1, 2, 3 and 4, representing adequate performance and mild, moderate, and severe impairment respectively. Postoperative scores were rated on the basis of 1 = no change, 2 = mild change, 3 = moderate change, and 4 = severe change. Productions were rated by two experienced examiners who achieved inter-rater reliability correlations of .69 (p < .01) for preoperative ratings and .43 (p < .05) for postoperative ratings. As an initial step in data assessment, the degree of preoperative impairment in performance was correlated with immediate postoperative change scores in such performance. In this instance a non-significant correlation co-efficient of + .36 was obtained. In effect, no significant relationship obtained here between the degree of preoperative impairment and the degree of postoperative change which may occur following either a VL or pulvinar lesion. On the other hand, a number of changes in Bender-Gestalt performance were noted when pre- to postoperative and pre- to long range changes were computed for both the pulvinar and ventrolateral lesion groups. Because of the small number of patients involved extensive statistical analysis was not undertaken. By observation, however, for pulvinar lesions it was noted that 6 of 14 patients manifested postoperative changes which may be described as mild or moderate, while for the ventrolateral lesion group 6 of 7 patients demonstrated changes rated as mild or moderate. In addition, no differences in the degree of changes scores were noted when left and right hemisphere operates were compared either for the pulvinar or VL lesion group. In the long range status both lesion groups had returned essentially to their preoperative stage, with 3 pulvinar patients manifesting mild postoperative changes and no patients in the VL group manifesting such change.

A small number (N = 9) of pulvinar operates had all or a portion of the Wechsler Memory Scale Form I administered pre- and immediately postoperatively. Only 2 of the subtests were altered postoperatively to any apparent degree. In the first instance the mean Digit Span score decreased 1.5 points, a confirmation of similar changes noted earlier on the Wechsler Adult Intelligence Scale. One other significant change was in visual reproduction in which a score increase from 7.2 to 9.6 occurred. This represents a rather significant improvement in a test of visual memory from pre- to post-operatively. However, it is based upon a rather small number of patients (N = 5) and only one showed a marked point increase in score. It is quite possible also that increments in such scores may represent a memory or practice effect since this test would seem to be susceptible to such effect. At any rate, it suggests, at least, that no apparent decrease in score obtained for pulvinar operates who were administered the test pre- and postoperatively.

Note should also be made of 4 patients who had combined pulvinar and VL lesions and for whom psychological test data are available. Unfortunately, none of these patients were fully testable (due to severe motor disabilities) and in most instances only the verbal portion of the standardized Intelligence Scale could be given. However, it is worthy of note that when pre- to postoperative mean scores were compared for these 4 patients the only subtest which altered pre- to postoperatively was the Digit Span in which a score reduction from 12.5 to 10.25 was noted, essentially comparable to changes previously observed for the pulvinar and ventrolateral groups individually. One is impressed, moreover, by the fact that the same overall change patterns as for the pulvinar and VL lesions occurred, at least with respect to verbal performance.

Another area worthy of comment concerns behavioral observations of the postoperative patients, other than those derived from specific test scores. In a preliminary report (Brown, Riklan, Waltz, Jackson, & Cooper, 1971), it was suggested that some of the early pulvinar lesion group of patients seemed to demonstrate what were described as "emotional" or behavioral changes. This kind of change was also previously noted by Kudo *et al.* (1968). Therefore, all of the patients in both pulvinar and ventrolateral groups, were observed on a daily basis following surgery, and both nurses' and doctors' notes were reviewed. In some instances patients clearly manifested alterations in behavioral lability or in intensity of emotional expression. For example, in 2 patients with preexisting left hemisphere lesions, increased depression and irritability and reduced emotional control was noted for several weeks following left pulvinectomy. In 2 other instances right pulvinectomy produced a reduction of "pathological crying" and emotional lability or explosiveness. This pattern of laterality may be of relevance. However, for the total sample now under consideration no clearcut pattern of alteration in emotional behavior or personality has been discernible. Indeed, in the vast majority of patients no observable emotional or behavioral change was noted in either direction. This finding held true particularly for patients such as dystonics and others whose preoperative brain, behavior, and emotional function was adequately intact and without structural damage. Changes noted earlier occurred primarily in patients with impaired brain and behavior functions including those having suffered strokes, brain concussion, and cerebral palsy.

## BILATERAL PULVINAR LESIONS

Three patients who underwent bilateral pulvinar surgery have had standardized pre- and postoperative cognitive and perceptual testing administered. Since this is too small a group to warrant statistical analysis, case reports and individual test findings are presented.

### Case # 1

T. Y. This is a 45-year old male with an 8-year history of torticollis which had progressed to a marked degree with

symptoms including severe pain, interfering with his function. The patient underwent a left cryopulvinectomy on June
10, 1971 and a right pulvinectomy on June 21. He was administered the Wechsler Adult Intelligence Scale 2 days prior to
his first operation, 8 days following this operation, 7 days
following the second operation, and again 4 months following
the second side surgery. Table 3 shows the WAIS scaled
subtest scores for this series of verbal and nonverbal performances.

TABLE 3
PRE AND POSTOPERATIVE SCALED WAIS SUBTEST SCORES FOR T.Y.

| Sub-Test | Preoperative 6/8/71 | Postoperative (L) 6/18/71 | 2nd Postoperative (R) 6/28/71 | Long Range Postoperative 10/27/71 |
|---|---|---|---|---|
| Information | 10 | 11 | 9 | 11 |
| Comprehension | 17 | 16 | 15 | 16 |
| Arithmetic | 13 | 12 | 11 | 14 |
| Similarities | 13 | 12 | 12 | 13 |
| Digit Span | 12 | 12 | 10 | 12 |
| Vocabulary | 11 | 11 | 10 | 11 |
| Digit Symbol | 5 | 5 | 4 | 14 |
| Picture Completion | 9 | 13 | 11 | 11 |
| Block Design | 10 | 12 | 10 | 7 |
| Picture Arrangement | 10 | 9 | 9 | 10 |
| Object Assembly | 10 | 13 | 12 | 10 |
| Verbal I.Q. | 118 | 116 | 109 | 119 |
| Performance I.Q. | 104 | 114 | 106 | 101 |
| Full-Scale I.Q. | 112 | 116 | 108 | 112 |

It is noted that no significant changes (except increments
due to possible practice effects) occurred from pre- to postoperatively following the initial left-sided lesion, and relatively small changes occurred immediately postoperatively
following the second side lesion. Furthermore, some 4 months
following second side surgery the patient's overall score had
returned essentially to its preoperative level. With respect
to specific subtests, a long range increase had occurred in
Digit Symbol performance, due possibly to improved motor
ability and a small decrease in Block Design performance,
possibly reflecting less integrated perceptual integration.
However, these individual subtests are not sufficiently reliable to warrant specific interpretations of these findings.

## Case # 2

M.O. is a 13-year old female with a 3-year history of Dystonia Musculorum Deformans. She was administered the Wechsler Intelligence Test for Children preoperatively, 7 days following a left cryopulvinectomy, 4½ months following left pulvinectomy, and 5 days following a right pulvinectomy. Table 4 shows the four sets of scores.

TABLE 4
PRE AND POSTOPERATIVE WISC SCALED SUBTEST SCORES FOR M.O.

| Sub-Test | Preaperative 6/16/71 | Postoperative (L) 6/24/71 | Long Range 11/1/71 | Postoperative (R) 11/15/71 |
|---|---|---|---|---|
| Information | 12 | 14 | 13 | 13 |
| Comprehension | 7 | 7 | 5 | 7 |
| Arithmetic | 10 | 9 | 10 | 12 |
| Similarities | 12 | 13 | 12 | 12 |
| Vocabulary | 13 | 12 | 10 | 11 |
| Digit Span | 16 | 14 | 12 | 14 |
| Picture Completion | 13 | 12 | 12 | 15 |
| Picture Arrangement | 8 | 5 | 13 | 5 |
| Block Design | 13 | 11 | 12 | 11 |
| Object Assembly | 7 | 11 | 6 | 7 |
| Coding | 12 | 5 | 11 | 6 |
| Verbal I.Q. | 113 | 110 | 103 | 110 |
| Performance I.Q. | 104 | 92 | 106 | 92 |
| Full-Scale I.Q. | 109 | 101 | 104 | 101 |

Immediately after left cryopulvinectomy decrements occurred primarily in performance I.Q. contributed largely by a reduction in Coding score. In longer range testing her scores had returned close to their preoperative level. Following a second side cryothalamectomy a small decrement was again noted during testing 14 days postoperatively. Again this decline seemed largely due to a reduction in the Coding subtest as well as a reduction in score on Picture Arrangement. As previously, individual subtest scores are not of sufficient reliability to draw definitive conclusions.

## Case # 3

N.T. is a 12-year-old right-handed girl who was admitted to the Neurosurgical Service with a history of severe progressive Dystonia Musculorum Deformans beginning at the age of 6. She had previously undergone a right cryothalamotomy (VL) in April of 1971 with some improvement. The Stanford-

Binet test was administered preoperatively and following left and right pulvinectomy with the following score findings: Preoperative left pulvinectomy (5/26/71)—102; immediate postoperative (6/7/71)—103; preoperative right pulvinectomy (11/3/71)—87; 14 days postoperatively (11/17/71)—87. It is noted that the patient was rather heavily medicated during the testing of 11/3/71, which may account for the decline in her test score. Retesting on 3/16/72 revealed an S-B I.Q. of 95, probably not significantly different from her preoperative baseline score of 102.

With respect to bilateral pulvinar lesions, it may tentatively be concluded that in subjects with no apparent pre-existing structural brain damage or evidence of behavioral or test deterioration, such lesions can be tolerated without significant lasting cognitive or perceptual alterations. The implications of this finding will be further considered in the discussion section.

## DISCUSSION

For the unilaterally placed pulvinar lesion, perhaps the most salient finding is for mean psychological test scores to show overall decrements immediately postoperatively, but with no specific change in the patterning of variability of such psychological functions as cognition, perception, memory, and perceptual-motor performance. A similar immediate postoperative decline occurred for a comparative sample of individuals undergoing VL surgery during the same time period. Moreover, this pattern of immediate postoperative decrements is remarkably similar to the postoperative changes previously reported following ventrolateral, globus pallidus, and subthalamic lesions for the relief of parkinsonian symptoms (McFie, 1960; Riklan, Diller, and Weiner, 1960; Jurko and Andy, 1964; Riklan and Levita, 1969). The similarity in patterning of postoperative declines between pulvinar, VL, and other subcortical lesion holds, furthermore, with respect to the specific subtests of psychological performance which are most vulnerable to such lesions, in particular Digit Span, and to a lesser degree Arithmetic and Digit Symbol. This particular pattern of decline appears to be rather nonspecific in nature and, as previously suggested, may be interpreted as representing "interference with the more immediate mobilization of mental energy" (Riklan *et al.*, 1960, p. 40) required for a variety of cognitive and perceptual functions, and particularly affects attention, concentration and recent memory. Such changes seem related more to temporary physiologic alterations in brain integration rather than to deficits specific to a particular lesion site.

Within the overall pattern of immediate postoperative decrements in a variety of psychological and behavioral functions, one special differentiation obtains. In particular, different degrees of postoperative alterations appear to result from left and right-sided lesions, whether the pulvinar or VL nucleus is involved. Specifically, patients undergoing left thalamic surgery decline more significantly in verbally mediated cognitive performance than those undergoing right-sided surgery. In contrast, no significant changes whatever, either in verbal or nonverbal tests, occurred in patients having undergone right hemisphere surgery. This finding would seem to confirm a number of earlier suggestions concerning a thalamic role either in language per se, or verbal test performance, and a lateralization of this function to the left hemisphere (cf, Penfield and Roberts, 1959; Riklan and Levita, 1969).

During over a decade of thalamic surgery for parkinsonism, numerous clinical investigators have noted immediate postoperative alterations in speech or language. Speech difficulties during the first two weeks after surgery were reported by Cooper (1961) for some 10% of patients undergoing unilateral chemopallidectomy and chemothalamectomy. About 20% of these were described as "aphasic", and this alteration was believed to follow operation on the dominant hemisphere, and to improve within several weeks. In contrast to unilateral intervention, bilateral basal ganglia surgery does seem to threaten "speech" in a more enduring manner. Indeed, among the first 100 consecutive patients with such operations, 18% experienced some transient speech abnormality, 6% having a lasting handicap, which simulated the speech of pseudobulbar palsy. A statistical tabulation of the sequelae for 1001 consecutive patients undergoing cryosurgery for parkinsonism (Waltz, Riklan, Stellar, and Cooper, 1966) indicated that "speech" deficits occurred immediately after surgery in 13.1% of patients. In the case of unilateral operations such deficits again were described as transient, with indications of more enduring alterations in the case of bilateral operates.

Similar observations have been reported elsewhere, although lack of consensual validation due to the absence of operational definitions, differences in surgical techniques, and questions of reliability concerning clinical impressions without adequate control limits the validity of comparisons between diverse groups. References to the literature are made with these limitations in mind. "A true disorder of language" of several weeks' duration was reported after left pallidal surgery in one study (Svennilson, Torvik, Lowe, and Leksell, 1960), while transient "dysphasia" for some patients following left hemisphere thalamic lesions was noted in another (Allan, Turner, and Gadea-Ciria, 1966). Hartmann-von Monakow (1965) also described disorders of expression, similar to cortically produced aphasia, in parkinsonians following diencephalic lesions. Such findings led Lennenberg (1967) to state that "the evidence is strong that speech and language are not confined to the cerebral cortex" (p. 64). In contrast, slurring and stuttering in the absence of a "true aphasia" was noted by others (Markham and Rand, 1963), following unilateral subcortical surgery of either hemisphere. After bilateral operations, slurring, dysarthria, and decreased volume were also reported by Krayenbuhl, Wyss, and Yasargil (1961). In addition, changes in vocalization, particularly in patterns of rate and rhythm, were observed following electrical stimulation of subcortical structures in the course of stereotaxic surgery, lending further credence to the possible role of these areas in verbal behaviors (Van Buren, 1963; Guiot, Hertzog, Rondet, and Molina, 1961; Schaltenbrand, 1965). Whether this role is purely motor in nature, e.g. articulation of symbols, or whether it involves the actual availability of verbal symbols is not yet clear.

Hermann, Turner, Gillingham, and Gaze (1966) assessed dysphasia, dysarthria, and voice volume in relation to stimulation and surgical lesions of the basal ganglia in parkinsonians. They found dysphasia occurred only after left-sided lesions in right-handed patients. The mean size of lesions in patients developing dysphasia was greater than the mean size of the total group studies. Furthermore, according to these authors pure capsular lesions did not result in dysphasia, suggesting a subcortical mechanism for this disturbance. Dysarthria also seemed more closely related to left hemisphere thalamic and globus pallidus lesions, and was particularly manifest following second hemisphere surgery. In bilateral operations, a right-sided lesion if added to a left-sided lesion produced dysarthria more commonly than when a left lesion was added to a right one. Finally, unilateral left-sided lesions appeared frequently to cause deterioration of voice volume whatever the preoperative status had been.

The verbally mediated psychological tests administered here were not selected to assess language and its alterations directly. However, the close relationship between the functions assessed by such batteries of tests and those involved in language and, consequently its impairment, was established previously (Reitan, 1954; Riklan, Diller, Weiner, and Cooper, 1960; Sklar, 1963; Piercy, 1964). The contents of present day tests of aphasia further illustrate this correspondence. For example, areas traditionally assessed by such tests include information, verbal comprehension, numerical ability, and concept formation (Head, 1926; Eisenson, 1954; Jones and Wepman, 1961; Schuell, Jenkins, and Jimenez-Pabon, 1964), and impairments in these areas have been identified with "reduction of vocabulary" by Schuell and Jenkins (1959, 1961). Moreover, a psycholinguistic analysis of 17 frequently used tests of aphasia (Osgood and Miron, 1963; Appendix B), shows that all deal with basic intellectual functions and processes. In this particular framework, "aphasic disorders may be viewed in most general form as the impairment of

intellectual functioning (Osgood and Miron, 1963, p. 176)".
Despite the narrower range of output assessed by psychological instruments, i.e., largely oral responses as distinguished
from reading, writing, and vocalization, required in aphasia
tests, it has been contended that "the same kind of linguistic
impairment tends to be apparent in all modalities" (Schuell,
Jenkins, and Jimenez-Pabon, 1964, p. 104).

The recent reports of Ojemann and his associates (1968,
1971a,b) in which stimulation of both the pulvinar and VL
thalamus on the left hemisphere resulted in altered ver-
balization, described as anomia by these authors, also lend
credence to a thalamic role, if not in the actual ability to
develop conceptualization and thinking through symbols,
then at least in the individual's ability to perform the motor
or expressive acts required to make such verbally mediated
responses. Whether the deficits in verbal performance or language functions during stimulation or following lesions in
thalamic nuclei represent indeed a "true aphasia" or perhaps
some form of perceptual or motor deficit remains for future
investigation to determine.

In the longer range situation, although only limited data
are now available, it would appear that mean scores for
patients, following either pulvinar or VL lesions, return essentially to their preoperative status, as did those previously
described for other series of VL and globus pallidus lesions
(Riklan and Levita, 1969). This finding may be related to
the fact that such surgical lesions ordinarily involve only portions of larger zones of functional activity, and that sufficient
mechanisms of neural duplication and replication are available so that no continuing functional deficit is manifest. As
an example, in postmortem studies of three patients previously subjected to pulvinectomy lesions were typically
described as including no more than one half of the nucleus,
or less (Cooper, 1972). A question may also be raised, however, as to whether current standardized psychological tests
are sufficiently refined to discern possible subtle continuing
changes which might result from such lesions. This may be.
However, the following possibilities are here suggested:

(1) compensatory mechanisms, plasticity or duplication of function within the thalamus or the hemisphere permit the re-establishment of integrated behavioral patterns so that no continuing deficits remain in functional performance;

(2) that alternate mechanisms utilizing the other hemisphere becomes available, or

(3) the particular functions being tested are not directly related to VL or pulvinar zones. Until further data are available, our hypothesis remains that, given time, integrated functions can emanate unimpaired following the delimited unilateral surgical lesions here under consideration, despite the fact that large numbers of neurons are destroyed.

With respect to psychological effects of bilateral pulvinar lesions, here as in the preliminary report of Brown, Riklan, and Cooper (1972), no evidence of marked impairment in cognitive, perceptual, or memory functions were noted either immediately postoperatively or in the long range testing, after a second sided lesion placed in the pulvinar. Moreover, in 2 of the 3 patients (both dystonics) with bilateral pulvinar lesions, two previous lesions had been placed in the VL thalamus. It is also worthy of note that in the past many patients with a diagnosis of Dystonia Musculorum Deformans have had three to six lesions placed in the thalamus, bilaterally, without any clinically apparent untoward effects in intellectual functions (Cooper, 1968).

With respect to bilateral subcortical lesions placed in several reported series of parkinsonians, and judging from results obtained through present testing of pulvinar operates, it would appear that such surgically induced lesions restricted to the globus pallidus, VL thalamus or pulvinar need have no significant lasting effect on cognitive-perceptual functions. Such a proposition corroborates the clinical findings reported previously by others (Gillingham, 1960–1961; Hassler and Reichert, 1958; Krayenbuhl, Wyss, and Yasargil, 1960; Krayenbuhl and Yasargil, 1961). Thus, while it is clinically apparent, and data on length of hospitalization confirm the fact, that second side thalamic surgery involves a longer and more arduous immediate postoperative course, a functional reorganization of "higher" integrative behavior seems to occur in due time.

The large size of the pulvinar, its development during recent phylogenetic stages, and its presumed connections with sensory areas of the cortex, particularly the temporal-parietal areas, and its possible connections with limbic structures raises the question as to its possible role in behavioral functions other than those generally termed cognitive and perceptual as tested with standardized tests. The observations of Kudo *et al.* (1968) of transient emotional effects in patients following pulvinectomy for pain is also relevant. Recent studies of Kreindler, Crighel and Marinchescu (1968) and Crighel and Kreindler (this monograph) also suggest that the pulvinar may participate both in sensory integration and modulation of cortical responses to various stimuli. And previously, Orchinik, Koch, Wycis, Fried and Spiegel (1949) had reported that dorsomedial thalamotomy reduced excessive fearfulness, apprehension and depression in some cases, with Spiegel, Wycis, Fried and Orchinik (1951–1952) including several thalamic nuclei in the neural systems related to emotional behavior. Consequently, it was of special interest that several patients, earlier in the unilateral pulvinar series, appeared to manifest behavioral or emotional changes in the area of "modulation" of behavior. As previously noted, 2 patients showed apparent increases in emotionality and agitation, while several others who tended, preoperatively, to be explosive and overemotional appeared to have this behavioral variable reduced and modulated somewhat. Some lateralization of this function was also suggested (Brown *et al.*, 1971). Consequently, such possible changes were carefully monitored in the remainder of the series. However, no specific pattern of modulation, increase, or reduction of emotional behavior, activation or emotional control was noted in most of the patients other than those seemingly related to symptomatic improvement or the lack thereof. Those few patients who manifested such alterations were in most instances individuals with pre-existing structural brain damage due to stroke, trauma, or injury. Consequently, it would now appear that in the essentially normally functioning brain with a normal resulting behavioral pattern, no apparent behavioral alterations result from the size and site of the lesions under consideration here. On the other hand, such lesions may exert some type of modulating effect in brains (and behavior) whose damage has resulted in untoward behavior in one or the other end of the emotional or activation scale. Further data are needed in this respect.

From the psychological test results and behavioral observations, the conclusion seems warranted that perhaps the overriding factor predictive of the types of psychological alterations which may result from thalamic lesions (pulvinar and VL) is the condition of the brain prior to such lesion production. It was noted in a preliminary report (Brown, Riklan, Waltz, Jackson, and Cooper, 1971) that individuals with unimpaired preoperative language and cognition can undergo unilateral right or left pulvinectomy without major alteration during the immediate postoperative period. That observation may now be extended to include a wider variety of cognitive, perceptual and motor functions in a larger series of patients, and would seem to obtain for bilateral as well as unilateral lesions. These findings also represent an extension of those made in a larger series of parkinsonians following ventrolateral thalamic surgery (Riklan and Levita, 1969). Previously, documentation was provided by Samra, Riklan, Levita, and Cooper (1971) in which pre- and postoperative psychological status of a series of patients with pathological confirmation of lesions were individually assessed. It was concluded then that the preoperative behavioral status rather than the specific site or size of the thalamic lesion was most crucial in determining whether psychological or behavioral alterations will occur postoperatively. Reinforcement of this observation comes from consideration of the somewhat larger deficits manifested by that sample of older parkinsonians, whose alterations tended to be somewhat greater following a VL lesion, as compared with the lesser alterations in the present series of younger pulvinar and VL lesion patients, which includes a large number of adolescents including dystonics. It is also demonstrated by individual case analyses in which dystonics, for example, seemed capable of sustaining two, three, or more VL and pulvinar lesions with apparent absence of untoward effect, when in contrast individuals with stroke or trauma tended to show greater postoperative deficits with similarly placed lesions.

Finally, the question arises concerning the role of the human thalamus generally, and its various nuclei, specifically in "higher" integrative behavioral functions. Data now exist with respect to effects of thalamic stimulation and/or lesion production in several different nuclei, in particular the ventrolateral nucleus, the dorsomedial nucleus, the centrum medianum, the ventroposterolateral, and the pulvinar, among others. It is also clear that thalamic nuclei participate in the processing and probably in the elaboration of most information eventually reaching the cortex. In addition, thalamocortical systems participate in a variety of "diffuse" activities which affect behavior (Jasper *et al.*, 1949, 1960). Therefore, most stimuli affecting and effecting behavior must involve thalamic structures. At the thalamic level a form of integration or processing of information occurs as it relates to extra and intraorganismic events. However, it is difficult to deduce, merely on the basis of small lesions placed in a portion of a thalamic nucleus, exactly the kind of functions involved, or even the kind of alterations which occur following such lesions, particularly since sufficient plasticity or flexibility appears to exist within the thalamus so that such lesions cause only temporary disruption. However, by considering some of these temporary disruptions, particularly in conguence with those caused by stimulations which result in an immediate effect, some concepts can be developed. On this basis, for example, it would seem that some aspects of language function somehow may be integrated in the thalamus. Indeed, one might conceive of the thalamus as a paradigm of the cortex, particularly with respect to sensory-motor integration. However, much further investigation, both in the laboratory and the clinic, is indicated before one can be more conclusive with respect to thalamic mechanisms of human psychological functions.

## References
Allan, C.M., Turner, T.W., and Gadea-Ciria, M.: Investigation into speech disturbances following stereotaxic surgery for parkinsonism. *Brit. J. Dis. Commun. 1:*55–59, 1966.

Brown, J.W., Riklan, M., Waltz, J.M., Jackson, S., and Cooper, I.S.: Preliminary studies of language and cognition following surgical lesions of the pulvinar in man (Cryopulvinectomy). *International J. Neurol. 8:*276–299, 1971.

Brown, J.W., Riklan, M., and Cooper, I.S.: Effects upon language and cognition of bilateral surgical lesions in human pulvinar. (Unpublished data)

Clark, W., LeGross, M., and Northfield, D.: The cortical projection of the pulvinar in the Macaque monkey. *Brain, 60:*126–142, 1927.

Cooper, I.S.: Personal Communications, 1972.

Cooper, I.S.: Role of the thalamus in motor function. Presented at Fulton Society, October 1971, Washington, D.C.

Cooper, I.S., Waltz, J.M., Amin, I., and Fujita, S.: Pulvinectomy: A preliminary report. *J. Amer. Geriatr. Soc. 19:*553–554, 1971.

Cooper, I.S.: *Involuntary Movement Disorders.* New York, Harper & Row, 1968.

Cooper, I.S.: *Parkinsonism: Its Medical and Surgical Therapy.* Springfield, Ill., Charles C Thomas, 1961.

Crighel, E., and Kreindler, A.: The role of the thalamic pulvinar-lateralis posterior complex in modulating neocortical reactivity. Presented at St. Barnabas Hospital Symposium, March 1972.

Eisenson, J.: *Examining for Aphasia.* New York, Psychological Corp., 1954.

Gillingham, J.: Surgical treatment of parkinsonism. *Trans. Med. Soc. London, 77:*52–56, 1960–1961.

Guiot, G., Hertzog, E., Rondet, T., and Molina, P.: Arrest of acceleration of speech evoked by thalamic stimulation in the course of stereotaxic procedures for parkinsonism. *Brain, 84:*363–379, 1961.

Hartmann-von Monakow, K.: Psychosyndrome und Sprachstoerungen nach stereotaktischen operationen beim Parkinson-Syndrom. *Akt. fragen. Psychiat. Neurol. 2:*87–100, 1965.

Hassler, R. and Reichert, T.: Ueber die symptomatik und operative behandlung der extrapyramidalen bewegungstoerungen. *Med. Klin. 53:*817–824, 1958.

Head, H.: *Aphasia and Kindred Disorders of Speech.* New York, Hafner. 1926.

Hermann, K., Turner, J.W., Gillingham, F.J., and Gaze, R.M.: The effects of destructive lesions and stimulation of the basal ganglia on speech mechanisms. *Cofin. Neurol. 27:*197–207, 1966.

Jasper, H.: Unspecific thalamo-cortical relations. In J. Field (Ed.) *Handbook of Physiology,* Section 1, Vol. II. Washington, D.C.: American Physiological Soc., pp. 1307–1322, 1960.

Jasper, H.: Diffuse projection systems: The integrative action of the thalamic reticular system. *Electroencephal. Clin. Neurophysiol. 1:*405–420, 1949.

Jones, L.V. and Wepman, J.M.: Dimensions of language performance in aphasia. *J. Speech Hearing Res. 4:*220–232, 1961.

Jurko, M.F. and Andy, O.J.: Psychological aspects of diencephalotomy. *J. Neurol. Neurosurg, Psychiat. 27:*516–521, 1964.

Krayenbuhl, H., Wyss, O.A.M. and Yasargil, M.G.: Bilateral thalamotomy and pallidotomy as treatment for bilateral parkinsonism. *J. Neurosurg. 18:*429–444, 1961.

Krayenbuhl, H. and Yasargil, M.G.: Ergebnisse der stereotakischen Operationen beim Parkinsonismus, insbesondere der doppelseitigen Eingriffe. *Deutsch Z. Nerven heilk, 182:*530–541, 1961.

Kreindler, A., Crighel, E., and Marinchescu, C.: Integrative activity of the pulvinar-lateralis posterior complex and interrelations with the neocortex. *Exper. Neurol. 22:*423–435, 1968.

Kudo, T., Yoshii, N., Shimizu, S., Aikawa, S., and Nishioka, S.: Stereotaxic thalamotomy for pain relief. *Tohuko Journal of Exper. Med. 96:*219–234, 1968.

Lennenberg, G.H.: *Biological Foundations of Language.* New York, Wiley, 1967.

McFie, J.: Psychological effects of stereotaxic operations for the relief of parkinsonian symptoms. *J. Ment. Sci. 106:*1512–1517, 1960.

Markham, C.H. and Rand, R.W.: Stereotactic surgery in Parkinson's Disease. *Neurology, 8:*621–631, 1963.

Meier, M.J. and Story, J.L.: Selective impairment of Porteus Maze test performance of the right subthalamotomy. *Neuropsychologia, 5:*181–189, 1967.

Ojemann, G., Fedio, P., and Van Buren, J.: Anomia from pulvinar and subcortical parietal stimulation. *Brain, 91:*99–116, 1968.

Ojemann, G., Blick, K.I., and Ward, A.A.: Improvement and disturbance of short-term verbal memory with human ventrolateral thalamic stimulation. *Brain, 94:*225–240, 1971.

Ojemann, G. and Ward, A.: Speech representation in ventrolateral thalamus. *Brain, 94:*669–680, 1971.

Osgood, C. and Miron, M.: *Approaches to the Study of Aphasia.* Urbana, Univ. Illinois Press, 1963.

Papez, J.: Connections of the pulvinar. *Arch. Neurol. Psychiat. 41:*277–289, 1939.

Penfield, W. and Roberts, L.: *Speech and Brain Mechanisms.* Princeton, Princeton University Press, 1959.

Perret, E. and Siegfried, J.: Memory and learning performance of parkinson patients before and after thalamotomy. In F. John Gillingham & I.M.L. Donaldson (Eds.) *Third Symposium on Parkinson's Disease.* Edinburgh, E. & S. Livingston, Ltd., pp. 164–168, 1969.

Piercy, M.: The effects of cerebral lesions on intellectual functions: A review of current research trends. *Brit. J. Psychol. 110:*310–352, 1964.

Reitan, R.M.: Intelligence and language functions in dysphasic patients. *Disease of the Nervous Systems, 15:*131–137, 1954.

Richardson, D.E.: Thalamotomy for intractable pain. Third International Symposium on Stereoencephalatomy, Madrid, 1967. *Confina Neurologica*, 29:139–145, 1967.

Richardson, D.E. and Zorub, D.S.: Sensory function of the pulvinar. Fourth Symposium Int. Soc. Res. Stereoencephalatomy. *Confin. Neurol.* 32:165–173, 1970.

Riklan, M., Diller, L., and Weiner, H.: A psychological study on the effect of chemosurgery of the basal ganglia in Parkinsonism. I. Intellectual functioning. *Arch. Gen. Psychiat.* 2:21–31, 1960.

Riklan, M. and Levita, E.: *Subcortical Correlates of Human Behavior: A Psychological Study of Basal Ganglia and Thalamic Surgery.* Baltimore, Williams & Wilkins, 1969.

Riklan, M., Levita, E., and Cooper, I.S.: Psychological effects of bilateral subcortical surgery for Parkinson's Disease. *J. Nerv. Ment. Dis. 141:*403–409, 1966.

Samra, K., Riklan, M., Levita, E., and Cooper, I.S.: Psychological correlates of anatomically verified thalamic lesions in parkinsonians.*J. Nerv. Ment. Dis. 152:*96–105, 1971.

Schaltenbrand, G.: The effects of stereotactic electrical stimulation in the depth of the brain. *Brain,* 88:835–840, 1965.

Schuell, H. and Jenkins, J.J.: The nature of language deficit in aphasia. *Psychol. Rev.* 66:45–67, 1959.

Schuell, H. and Jenkins, J.J.: Reduction of vocabulary in aphasia. *Brain,* 84:243–246, 1961.

Schuell, H., Jenkins, J.J., and Jimenez-Pabon, E.: *Aphasia in Adults: Diagnosis, Prognosis, and Treatment.* New York, Harper & Row, 1964.

Simpson, D.: The projection of the pulvinar to the temporal lobe.*J. Anat.* 86:20–29, 1952.

Sklar, M.: Relation of psychological and language test scores and autopsy findings in aphasia. *J. Speech Hearing Res.* 6:84–90, 1963.

Spiegel, E.A., Wycis, H.T., Freed, H., and Orchinik, C.: The central mechanism of the emotions(experiences with circumscribed thalamic lesions). *Amer. J. Psychiat. 108:*426–432, 1951–1952.

Svennilson, E., Torvik, A., Lowe, R., and Leksell, L.: Treatment of parkinsonism by stereotactic thermolesions in the pallidal region. *Acta. Psychiat. Scand. 35:*358–377, 1960.

Truex, R. and Carpenter, M.: *Human Neuroanatomy.* Baltimore, Williams & Wilkins, 1969.

Van Buren, J.M.: Confusion and disturbance of speech from stimulation in vicinity of the head of the caudate nucleus.*J. Neurosurg. 20:*148–157, 1963.

Walker, A.E.: *The Primate Thalamus.* Chicago, The University of Chicago Press, 1928.

Walker, A.E.: The Thalamus. In D. Purpura and M. Yahr (Eds) *Internal Structure and Afferent-Efferent Relations of the Thalamus.* New York, Columbia University Press, pp. 1–12, 1966.

Waltz, J.M., Riklan, M., Stellar, S., and Cooper, I.S.: Cryothalamectomy for Parkinson's Disease: A statistical analysis. *Neurology,* *16*:994–1002, 1966.

# CHAPTER 7

# SPEECH AND SHORT-TERM VERBAL MEMORY

# ALTERATIONS EVOKED FROM STIMULATION IN PULVINAR

GEORGE A. OJEMANN, M.D.

THIS PAPER REVIEWS some changes in performance on a standard test of object naming and short-term verbal recall evoked by electrical stimulation of sites in anterior-superior pulvinar. These studies were carried out on patients undergoing stereotaxic procedures as part of the treatment for dyskinesias. The major findings in this review have been previously published (Ojemann, Fedio and Van Buren, 1968; Ojemann and Fedio, 1968). These studies were originally directed at relating ventrolateral thalamic structures to speech processes. In the particular stereotaxic technique that Dr. John Van Buren* used at that time, a multicontact depth electrode was chronically implanted with its deepest portion, containing a coagulating slug, in a target low in the ventrolateral thalamic nucleus (Van Buren, 1965a,b). The electrode was inserted either through a frontal or parietal burrhole. Rather unexpectedly, the most notable changes in performance on the standard test of object naming and short-term verbal memory were evoked from some of the electrode contacts lying some distance proximal to the coagulating slug in electrodes inserted through a parietal approach. Subsequent analysis suggested that these electrode contacts fell

---

* Surgical Neurology Branch, National Institutes of Health, Bethesda, Md. 20014.

within the anterior-superior corner of the pulvinar. Our publications were based on an earlier series of patients that has subsequently been expanded by Dr. Paul Fedio* and Dr. Van Buren. This paper will include the data on both the original and expanded series. Although the addition of further patients has given us the security of presenting larger numbers, it has not notably altered the findings originally published.

## METHODS

The detailed methodology used in these studies is described in the previous publications (Ojemann, Fedio and Van Buren, 1968; Ojemann and Fedio, 1968). Briefly, several days following implantation of the chronic multicontact depth electrode, the patient was trained and tested on the standard test of object naming presented on a screen via a Graflex projector controlled by an automatic timing device. The test consisted of chromatic pictures of a series of objects whose names are words of common frequency with the word "and" printed on a slide interspersed between slides picturing each object. The test is presented continuously. As the test initially begins, the patient names the object, reads the word "and" when it appears, then when the next object appears names it and gives the name of the object which appeared previous to the distraction provided by the "and". The sequence of this test is well-illustrated in Fedio and Weinberg (1971). Each object and the word "and" were presented for 4 seconds. After the patient had been performing the test for a variable period of time, bipolar stimulation of a pair of contacts, 5 mm. apart on the depth electrode, was undertaken using 12 second trains of 60 per second, 2½ ms duration biphasic square wave pulses from a constant current stimulator. The stimulus was always applied just at the beginning of the presentation of a new object; thus each stimulus encompassed the two objects to be named and the intervening picture of the word "and". The test was interrupted a number of objects after the end of the stimulus and the patient was interrogated as to whether he had felt anything. If sensations were evoked, that stimulation was discarded from further analysis.

EEG from adjacent electrode contacts and scalp was monitored during the course of stimulation and any trials on which
afterdischarges were evoked were discarded. All of the data
was recorded on multichannel magnetic tape. Electrode location was determined by measuring the location of each contact
on the electrode to the anterior or posterior commissure,
whichever was closer, the intercommissural line and the midline of the brain. Dr. Van Buren has a series of charts showing
the mean location and range of variation of the lateral thalamic
border and a number of structures within the thalamus including the central median-interlaminus nucleus and the pulvinar,
about these commissural reference points (Van Buren, 1972).
The midpoint between two electrode contacts stimulated was
plotted on these charts. If the midpoint fell medial to the
innermost range of variation of the lateral border of the
thalamus, that electrode contact pain was considered to lie
within the thalamus and was included in our analysis.

## ALTERATIONS IN EVOKED OBJECT NAMING

We established a number of definitions of the changes in
object naming that were evoked by stimulation. This discussion will be confined to only one type which we will call
"anomia". We defined anomia as the inability to name the
object, either an omission of the name or a misnaming, while
there was demonstrated retained ability to speak, such as
the patients being able to read "and" when it appeared on
the appropriate slide. We were particularly interested in this
type of object naming error, because in Penfield and Robert's
(1959) extensive review of the effects of cortical stimulation
on speech, it is this type of error which correlates most closely
with the cortical areas usually considered to subserve speech
and language function. Thus, this type of alteration in object
naming is evoked only from the dominant hemisphere, in
the third-frontal convolution (Broca's speech area), the region
of the angular and supramarginal gyri (the Wernicke speech
area) and from the supplementary motor area (on the medial
face of the hemisphere). Specifically, in Penfield and Robert's
data, the "anomic" type of response was not evoked from

the nondominant hemisphere nor from the motor strip of dominant or nondominant hemispheres.

The object naming test was quite easy for our patients in the absence of stimulation. Anomic errors occurred so rarely under these control conditions that the probability is very small that any such error of object naming evoked by stimulation is due to chance.

We found that when the electrodes had been inserted through a parietal burrhole to the target area low in the ventrolateral thalamus, the only site likely within the thalamus from which anomia was evoked was a cluster of electrode contacts lying medial to the most medial border of the range of variation of the lateral thalamic border, posterior to a coronal plane 3 mm. anterior to the posterior commissure, lateral to a parasagittal plane 12½ mm. lateral to the midline and superior to a horizontal plane, 7½ mm. above the intercommissural plane. In the initial published series (Ojemann, Fedio and Van Buren, 1968) there were 8 patients with electrode contacts in this portion of left thalamus, in 5 of them anomic errors were evoked (including all the right-handed patients with stimulation currents at, or above, the smallest current evoking anomia). Seven patients had electrode contacts similarly placed in the right lateral thalamus; in only one of these (a left-handed patient) was anomia evoked. The difference in performance between this portion of right and left thalamus was statistically significant. This series has now grown to the point where it can be restricted to only right-handed patients. Doctors Fedio and Van Buren (personal communications, 1972) have kindly supplied me with this more recent data; it has been presented before (Ojemann, Fedio and Van Buren, 1969) but not published. There are now 13 right-handed patients with electrode contacts in this portion of the left posterior-superior lateral thalamus. Anomia has been evoked in 10 of them. Twelve right-handed patients have electrode contacts in this portion of right posterior-superior lateral thalamus; anomia has been evoked in *none* of them. Both the frequency of evoking anomia from this site in left thalamus, and the differential effect of left and right brain stimulation at this site are statistically highly significant.

Patients in the expanded series with electrodes in left or right pulvinar are comparable as to age (mean: left 45, right 48); ratio of males to females; I.Q. (mean: left 114, right 108); and memory quotient (mean: left 111, right 101). The average stimulating current is also comparable on the two sides, 5.1 ma. in the left and 4.9 ma. in the right, as is the average number of trials for each patient.

When the arbitrary coordinants that delimit the location of those electrode contacts with evoked anomia were compared to the anterior border of the range of variation of the pulvinar as determined by Dr. Van Buren, it was found that the two showed remarkable correspondence (see Ojemann, Fedio and Van Buren, 1968) for the electrode contact locations and line drawings of the range variation of the pulvinar nucleus. Thus, it appears that it is a portion of the anterio-superior pulvinar which is the location from which anomia has been so consistently evoked from the left side.

Histologic confirmation of this location was obtained in one case who succumbed to a massive right intracerebral hemorrhage some 3 weeks after left thalamic stimulation (and 3 days following right thalamic coagulation). The reconstruction of the actual location of that left thalamic electrode has been published in Ojemann, Fedio and Van Buren (1968), and the contacts between which stimulation evoked anomia were found to lie in the anterio-superior portion of the pulvinar. Electrode pairs immediately deep and immediately superficial to the pair from which anomia was evoked showed no alterations in object naming with stimulation.

Further evidence that pulvinar stimulation appears to alter object naming was obtained by determining the latency for object naming when stimulating currents were below the threshold for evoking anomia. Under these circumstances the average latency response was found to lengthen noticeably during stimulation of the electrode contacts in the anterio-superior portion of the left pulvinar, but not from the right (Ojemann, Fedio and Van Buren, 1968).

The threshold for evoking anomia from left pulvinar is relatively high, with a mean of 7.6 milliamps and a range from 4 to 14 milliamps in the initial series. The types of object naming errors made were mixed; approximately half the errors being misnamings, the remainder omissions. Anomia could be evoked on about ¾ of the successive stimulations in the same pair of electrode contacts at the same or larger currents.

## ALTERATIONS IN SHORT-TERM VERBAL MEMORY

During our standard test we asked the patient, once he had named the particular object showing on the screen, to also give us the name of the object immediately preceding, separated from this object by the 4-second distraction of the word "and" (Fedio and Weinberg, 1971). Analysis of this performance of the ability to recall the name of the previously presented object provides some measure of performance on short-term verbal memory. This analysis was restricted to current levels less than those interfering with object naming. It was also restricted to stimulations where the latency of object naming was less than 3 seconds, so as to provide an adequate amount of time for recall to occur. (Mean latencies of object naming are, in fact, 1.1 seconds (left) and 1.6 seconds (right) so that more than half of the 4 seconds exposure period is generally available for recall.)

Analyzing the effects of stimulation of electrode contacts in the same anterio-superior portion of pulvinar (considered to lie in that part of lateral thalamus bounded by the same arbitrary coronal plane 3 mm. anterior to the posterior commissural plane, the parasagittal plane 12½ mm. lateral to the midline and horizontal planes 7½ mm. above the intercommissural plane) shows a striking deterioration of recall performance when stimulation occurred in patients with left brain electrodes while there was no change in recall performance in patients with electrodes in right brain—a statistically significant differential effect. The initial series of patients in these groups have been published in Ojemann and Fedio (1968). Figure 1 demonstrates the data on the expanded series of patients. As in the initial portion of this series, stimulation

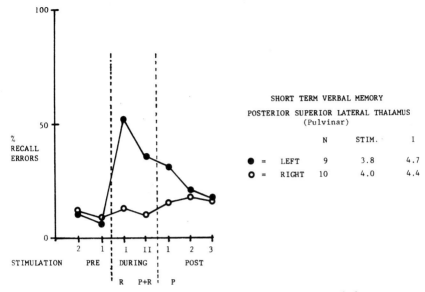

Figure 7-1. Mean percentage of recall errors at the time of objects presented before (pre 2, 1), during (I, II) and after (Post 1, 2, 3) stimulation in left and right pulvinar. N represents the number of patients with electrode contracts in either left or right pulvinar, Stm. the mean number of stimulations for each of these groups and I, the mean stimulating current level in milliamps for each group.

has a different effect on recall during the first or second object during stimulation. Recall performance is quite severely disturbed at the time of the first object during stimulation, and appreciably less disturbed at the time of the second object. Recall occurring at the time of the first object during stimulation is for material presented prior to stimulation. Another way of looking at this is that stimulation occurs during retrieval of information which is presented in the absence of stimulation (R on Figure 1). Recall at the time of the second object during stimulation is for material both presented and retrieved during stimulation (P + R on Figure 1). Recall at the time of the first object after stimulation is for material presented during stimulation and retrieved in the absence of stimulation (P on Figure 1). Stimulation of the electrode contacts in the left anterio-superior pulvinar particularly disturbs retrieval of information presented in the absence of stimulation. This effect is statistically significant even in the initial series (Ojemann and Fedio, 1968). Retrieval of information presented and retrieved during stimulation of these electrodes or material presented during stimulation but retrieved in the absence of stimulation are less seriously disturbed.

A partial explanation for this phenomenon became apparent following a study of the effects of stimulation in a more anterior portion of left lateral thalamus—the ventrolateral thalamic nucleus—on a somewhat different test of short-term verbal memory in which the input and retrieval functions were more readily separated (Ojemann, Blick, and Ward, 1971). Left ventrolateral thalamic stimulation during presentation was associated with an improvement in recall performance compared to nonstimulation control performance, an effect we attributed to an evoked direction of attention to verbal material present in the external environment. Stimulation during retrieval alone was associated with a marked deterioration in performance, and stimulation during both presentation and retrieval, performance was not different from control levels. It appears that in the pulvinar the effect associated with disturbance of retrieval with stimulation during retrieval alone is quite marked. The effect associated with direction of attention to verbal material present in the external environment during stimulation is also present, likely accounting for the fewer recall errors on the second object presented during stimulation. However, this effect is diminished in pulvinar, compared to more anteriorly in dominant lateral thalamus so that while with stimulation during presentation and retrieval, or presentation alone, performance improves over stimulation during retrieval alone, it does not improve to or over control levels (as it does in ventrolateral thalamus).

Thus, it appears that the dominant anterio-superior pulvinar in addition to showing evoked changes in object naming, that suggest that it participates in ideational speech mechanisms, also participates in retrieval mechanism of short-term verbal memory. Thus, there seems to be an overlap of speech and at least short-term verbal memory function in the anterio-superior pulvinar. Indeed, the anomic speech errors may represent a retrieval deficit, though involving long term rather than short-term verbal memory.

## RELATION OF EFFECTS OF PULVINAR STIMULATION TO EFFECTS OF PULVINAR LESIONS

As mentioned at the beginning of the paper, our data was derived from electrode contacts "en passage" to a target area in ventrolateral thalamus. Coagulations were not carried out in the area of pulvinar sampled by our electrodes. Thus, we have no direct data on the effects of lesions in this area on the tests of object naming and short-term verbal memory that we have used. It is even rather difficult to speculate on what one might expect to see from such lesions. In a recently published paper, Ojemann and Ward (1971) reported that anomia was evoked from a discrete medial central area of dominant ventrolateral thalamic nucleus. Lesions in dominant ventrolateral thalamus give rise to a transient anomia rather frequently. In one series (Selby, 1967) this reaches 40 percent of patients, but permanently detectable speech deficits are rather rare from these lesions. Perhaps this is the same phenomenon that Penfield and Roberts (1959) observed in comparing the effects on speech of cortical lesion and stimulation. They report relatively small lesions placed in portions of cortex that seem to subserve ideational speech function (as determined by stimulation) will give rise to a transient but not necessarily a permanent anomia, while large lesions in the same area generally give permanent anomia. Whether the speech deficit is permanent or not, is more a function of the size of the lesion within the speech area, and the adequacy of function of the remaining areas that subserve speech function rather than the exact location of the lesion alone. The pulvinar is also a very large nucleus, and it well may be that stimulation and lesions in different areas of pulvinar will have marked functional differences.

At the cortical level, the anomic type of error with stimulation during object naming seems to provide fairly accurate correlation with those parts of cortex where lesions will at least transiently produce alterations in ideational speech function (Penfield and Roberts, 1959). If the same analogy holds for subcortex, and to some extent it seems to for ventrolateral thalamus, then it seems likely that the lesion in or adjacent to the anterio-superior portion of the pulvinar will at least transiently disturb ideational speech function. Indeed, Ciemins (1970) reports such a case with a lesion involving the lateral aspect of the left lateral posterior nucleus, the left ventroposterior nucleus, and the medial third of the left pulvinar which was associated with prolonged aphasia. Penfield and Roberts (1959, p. 215) allude to a similar case.

There is less information on the effects of focal lesion of the human brain on short-term verbal memory. Short-term verbal memory can be disturbed after ventrolateral thalamic lesions acutely (Ojemann, Hoyenga and Ward, 1971) and occasionally even on a long-term basis (Krayenbuhl *et al.*, 1965). Verbal memory can also be altered after left temporal lobe lesions, the deficit increasing with more extensive hippocampal complex or lateral temporal involvement (Milner, 1967). Evidence that the anterio-superior pulvinar has an anatomical relationship with the lateral temporal lobe, and the adjacent parietal lobe is available (see Van Buren and Yakovlev, 1959; Van Buren and Borke, 1969). Thus, there seems to be an anatomic basis for anterio-superior pulvinar participation in ideational speech mechanism, and the same anatomic paths may subserve anterio-superior pulvinar and lateral temporal lobe short-term verbal memory functions. However, preliminary data on the effects of stimulation of the temporal-parietal speech area on short-term verbal memory have been conflicting (Fedio and Van Buren, 1971; Ojemann, unpublished data).

The study of the effects of electrical stimulation on tests of object naming and short-term verbal memory suggests that both of these functions are represented in the anterio-superior portion of the dominant pulvinar. From other portions of the dominant lateral thalamus changes in speech and short-term verbal memory can also be evoked, specifically, anomia can be evoked from the medial and central portions of ventrolateral thalamus (Ojemann and Ward, 1971) and short-term verbal memory changes throughout ventrolateral thalamus with characteristics which set ventrolateral thalamus somewhat apart from the changes evoked from pulvinar (Ojemann, Blick and Ward, 1971). Together these data suggest roles for dominant lateral thalamic structures in various higher intellectual functions.

The pulvinar connections with the anterio-temporal lobe and adjacent parietal lobe have been well discussed today. I think the evidence certainly seems to provide the anatomic basis for the anterio-superior pulvinar participation in ideational speech mechanism. The same anatomic pathway may subserve anterio-superior and lateral pulvinar and lateral temporal lobe short-term verbal memory functions.

Unfortunately, the study of short-term verbal memory functions in parietal cortex is still in its infancy and the initial data is somewhat conflicting.

## References

Ciemens, V.: Localized thalamic hemorrhage: a cause of aphasia. *Neurology*, *20*:776–782, 1970.

Fedio, P. and Van Buren, J.: Cerebral Mechanisms for Perception and Immediate Memory under Electrical Stimulation in Conscious Man. In Symposium: Human Memory: Cortical and Subcortical Mechanisms. Presented at Annual Meeting of American Psychological Association, Washington, D.C., 1971.

Fedio, P. and Weinberg, L.: Dysnomia and impairment of verbal memory following intracarotid injection of sodium amytal. *B. Research*, *31*:159–168, 1971.

Krayenbuhl, H., Siegfried, J., Kohenof, M., *et al.*: Is there a dominant thalamus? *Conf. Neurol. 26*:246–249, 1965.

Ojemann, G., Blick, K., and Ward, A.: Improvement and disturbance of short-term verbal memory with human ventrolateral thalamic stimulation. *Brain, 94*:225–240, 1971.

Ojemann, G. and Fedio, P.: Effect of stimulation of the human thalamus and parietal and temporal white matter on short-term memory. *J. Neurosurg. 29*:51–59, 1968.

Ojemann, G., Fedio, P., and Van Buren, J.: Anomia from pulvinar and subcortical parietal stimulation. *Brain, 91*:99–116, 1968.

Ojemann, G., Fedio, P., and Van Buren, J.: Evidence for dominance within the human lateral thalamus. 9th Int. Congress of Neurology. *Excerpta Medica Int. Congress Series, 193*:260 (abstract), 1969.

Ojemann, G., Hoyenga, K., and Ward, A.: Predictions of short-term verbal memory disturbance after ventrolateral thalamotomy. *J. Neurosurg.* 35:203–210, 1971.

Ojemann, G. and Ward, A.: Speech representation in ventrolateral thalamus. *Brain,* 94:669–680, 1971.

Penfield, W. and Roberts, L.: *Speech and Brain Mechanisms.* Princeton, Princeton University Press, 1959.

Selby, G.: Stereotaxic surgery for the relief of Parkinson's Disease. II. An analysis of the results of a series of 303 patients (413 operations). *J. Neurol. Sci.,* 5:343–375, 1967.

Van Buren, J.: Incremental Coagulation. In E. Spiegel *et al.* (Eds.) *Parkinson's Disease. Trends in Research and Treatment.* New York, Gruen & Stratton, 1965a.

Van Buren, J.: A stereotaxic instrument for man. *EEG Clin. Neurophysl.* 19:398–403, 1965b.

Van Buren, J.: *Variations of the Human Diencephalon,* Vol. II. Heidelberg, Springer-Verlag, 1972.

Van Buren, J. and Borke, R.: Alterations in speech and the pulvinar—A serial section study of cerebrothalamic relationships in cases of acquired speech disorders. *Brain,* 92:255–284, 1969.

Van Buren, J. and Yakovlev, P.: Connections of the temporal lobe in man. *Act. Anat.* 39:1–50, 1959.

## DISCUSSION

**Dr. Cooper:** Thank you, Dr. Ojemann. This has been a very stimulating paper.

**Dr. Van Buren:** I wondered if I could introduce one word of caution, along with this presentation. When we speak of aphasia we are speaking of a specific test which Dr. Ojemann has outlined for you: the ability to name an object, say the word and name the next object and recall it. And I would like to just read one response of a patient Dr. Fedio and I were working with a week before last, which I think is rather interesting. I am going to use the words 'non-stimulus presentation', 'non-stimulus response' and 'stimulus presentation' and 'stimulus response'. This is a non-stimulus presentation. It was a handsaw. Patient's response is "saw" and she sees hand and says "and".

Then we have a stimulus presentation of a tie. She says "tie" "saw" and then she gives the word "and" also during the stimulation. Then during the stimulation still she has the word "radio". She says "camera" and then "saw". In other words she has seen an object and misnamed it. And she is capable of saying the word "and". And she can remember what is given before. In another response she used the word "fox" for "squirrel". She was an intelligent lady, being operated on for torticollis. Now this is a nice aphasic response. The localization of the electrodes, however, is in the caudate head. Now this is something which Dr. Ojemann, Dr. Fedio and I had considered well before.

This is a study we made earlier of the response of the caudate and striatum, frontal striatal region, to stimulation and this was what we call the arrest response. It is a very curious thing. It stops speech, it stops any activity, it is not localized to the left hemisphere, and it can appear on both sides. There is post-stimulation confusion and inappropriate speech may be part of it. I won't bother with the rest of this, but I'm just bringing this up as a caution in evaluating aphasic responses. In other words, here is quite a different thing. During this post-stimulation confusion you may get garbled speech, peculiar speech, loss of orientation, and things of this sort.

The way this was controlled in the pulvinar study was to apply a test of continuous performance, which Dr. Mersky had devised for evaluating the level of consciousness during petit mal attacks. In other words, subjects were presented with a series of letters, about 25 percent X's, and when they had an X, they were supposed to press a key.

The difference between the caudate stimulations which gives this "aphasic" response and the pulvinar stimulations with the "aphasic" response is that the continuous performance test showed that the person with a caudate or striatal response was indeed turned off, if you like. It is a poor expression but I don't know what else to say. He was not responding or he could be confused, and he would forget to punch his key. Conversely, the person stimulated in the pulvinar would punch his key even though he couldn't get the word out, and there was a statistically significant difference between the responses. So I think, this is just a word of caution which we all have to think about as to whether we have something which actually interferes with speech itself or whether this is in part interference with the attention mechanism.

**Dr. Ojemann:** Let me add one comment to those of Dr. Van Buren. The "anomic response", as we defined it here, applies to some one who demonstrates during stimulation that he can speak; he simply can't name the required object. We have the same thing in this example.

## INVITED DISCUSSION
### Observations on Language Following Cryopulvinectomy
#### Dr. Brown

In the past year I have studied a series of patients undergoing cryopulvinectomy and have been concerned rather less with the effects of stimulation in the pulvinar than with the results of surgical lesion (cryopulvinectomy). In our initial report (Brown *et al.*, 1971) 10 cases of unilateral pulvinectomy and 1 case of bilateral pulvinectomy were described. Since this time, I have had the oppurtunity to examine approximately 20 additional unilateral cases, and three bilateral cases, and our subsequent studies have tended to confirm our initial impression.

With regard to the unilateral procedure it may interest you to know that this operation was initially carried out in the hope of finding a surgical treatment for severe aphasia. The observation by Dr. Cooper of a salutory effect in some cases of increased motor tone, led to the application of the procedure to the treatment of dystonia. This experience is reflected in Table 1 which summarizes our initial experience with this operation. I would like to call your attention to the wide age and even sex distribution and the fact that the initial cases were those of brain-damaged aphasic adults. As the operation was extended to dystonia, it was initially performed in the most severe cases, many with previous thalamic surgery.

Subjects with normal preoperative language and cognitive function, and particularly in the absence of structural brain damage, showed no evidence of aphasia or dementia following cryopulvinectomy in the speech-dominant hemisphere.

**TABLE 1**

| Case Number | Sex | Age | Diagnosis | Pulvinar Lesion Side | Handedness | Previous Thalamic Surgery |
|---|---|---|---|---|---|---|
| 1 | M | 71 | CVA, right hemiplegia, aphasia | left 4/22/71 right 5/5/71 | right | none |
| 2 | M | 39 | Cranial trauma, right hemiplegia, aphasia | left 4/29/71 | right | none |
| 3 | M | 51 | Cranial trauma, right hemiplegia, mild aphasia | left 5/3/71 | right | none |
| 4 | F | 11 | Dystonia musculorum deformans | left 5/27/71 | right | right thalamectomy 4/30/71 |
| 5 | M | 33 | Double athetosis | left 5/28/71 | right | left thalamectomy 7/30/66 right thalamectomy 7/9/70 |
| 6 | F | 13 | Dystonia musculorum deformans | left 6/17/71 | ambidextrous | left thalamectomy 10/15/70 right reinsertion 1/20/71 |
| 7 | F | 22 | Dystonia musculorum deformans | left 5/26/71 (VL) | right | left thalamectomy 2/2/62 right thalamectomy 6/5/62 |
| 8 | M | 45 | Torticollis | left 6/10/71 right 6/21/71 | left | none |
| 9 | F | 41 | Cerebral Palsy | right 6/16/71 | right | none |
| 10 | F | 10 | Dystonia musculorum deformans | left 6/21/71 | right | left thalamectomy 5/22/70 right thalamectomy 9/22/70 |
| 11 | M | 34 | Cerebral Palsy, choreoathetosis of left arm | right 7/1/71 | right | right chemothalamectomy 1/12/61 right reinsertion 2/13/61 |

However, some patients showed an immediate postoperative decrement in verbal learning as determined by such tests as supra-span word recall and paired associates. There was no indication that verbal material learned prior to surgery was affected by the operation. Mild reduction in digit span was also noted. In a few patients with pre-existing structural lesion and with borderline language or cognitive function, cryopulvinectomy in the dominant hemisphere did induce further deterioration. Of the 30 or so unilateral patients that we have seen thus far, there are only three instances, all with prior brain damage, of such deterioration. However, in the more optimal surgical group, the dystonics, the majority of whom had normal or above average I.Q. and intact language function, no deterioration in language was observed. We might emphasize, parenthetically, that such aphasic phenomena as have been observed, as in the above cases, consisted largely of anomic or misnaming states, and did not suggest the "cortical" syndromes of Wernicke's aphasia, conduction, or Broca's aphasia. Moreover, in all patients, speech comprehension appeared to be remarkably resistent.

We have also studied 3 cases of bilateral cryopulvinectomy. The pertinent features of these patients are summarized in Table II.

A mild decrement occurred on supra-span verbal recall, with an average reduction of two items per trial over 4 trials but good retention of words given prior to surgery. Slight decrement on digit span testing was also found, but bedside

TABLE 2

| Case | Sex | Age | Hand. | Diag. | Previous Surgery | Pulvinar Surgery |
|------|-----|-----|-------|-------|------------------|------------------|
| 1 | F | 13 | L | DMD | RVL(1970) LVL(1970) RVL(1971) | Left (6/71) Right (11/71) |
| 2 | F | 12 | R | DMD | RVL(1971) | Left (5/71 Right (11/71) |
| 3 | M | 45 | L | Torticollis | None | Left (6/10/71) Right (6/21/71) |

tests of memory were normal. Complete aphasia testing in all three patients demonstrated no abnormalities in speech, comprehension, naming, repetition, reading, writing, or spatial-constructional performance. In one case there was a slight tendency toward miniaturization on drawing, and occasional misspelling.

Certainly, we were surprised to find so little alteration in language following pulvinectomy, having anticipated from previous reports, some of which have been discussed here this morning, that the pulvinar might play a role in linguistic processes. And yet, it would seem that the pulvinar must play some role in linguistic or cognitive function. In the course of studying several patients with VL thalamotomy it was striking how similar the alterations of "higher function" were to those of pulvinectomy. This was brought out convincingly by Dr. Riklan earlier in the day. It seems that although large thalamic lesions may produce some language deterioration in an otherwise normally functioning brain, the effect of these lesions follows a kind of mass action. Thus, a patient with pre-existing structural brain damage or with borderline mental function may show regression after a single and even relatively small thalamic lesion. I suspect this explains the occurrence of such deficits following VL thalamotomy since the majority of patients were Parkinsonian. I think we would all agree that many patients with Parkinson's disease are functioning at a borderline mental level to begin with and have widespread pathology, and for this reason are obviously a less ideal patient group than the dystonics. This suggests that the effect of thalamic lesion, whether in VL or pulvinar, or perhaps in other nuclear groups as well, is to produce a mild regression which, in a relatively normal brain, is not sufficient to be clinically measured. However, in the presence of pre-existing borderline function, the regression then brings the patient into the sphere of the pathological. Still further regression would permit linguistic impairment to become testable. In this respect, it might be emphasized that those deficits which can be identified with thalamic lesion, namely anomic, verbal paraphasic, and verbal amnesic disorders, concern early stages in the cognitive-linguistic process. Significantly, these deep-level disorders are among the first to appear with generalized brain involvements or with focal damage outside the classical speech area.

Regarding the paper by Dr. Ojemann, I don't pretend to be able to resolve the difference in the findings reported upon stimulation in VL and anterior pulvinar, and those which I have described following pulvinectomy. I do believe there are certain problems arising in Dr. Ojemann's methodology which will require some clarification before his results can be fully accepted. I think the question of impaired visual discrimination should not be dismissed so lightly. Bisiach (1966) has demonstrated this to be an important factor even in standard *cortical* anomics. Perhaps a comparison of performance on objects of similar morphology might be of value. Moreover, it has to be emphasized that the naming of object pictures is perhaps the most challenging of naming tasks from the visual standpoint. These results should be compared with the naming of real objects. This objection could be overcome quite simply by asking the patients to name objects from description. Certainly, it should be correlated with performance on other modalities, such as naming objects by sound, touch, etc. Along this line, I would suggest a method which might disclose whether the patient is unable to *produce* or *pronounce* the word. Rather than have patients say a word like "and" to guarantee speech ability, perhaps they might be requested to preface each name by phrases such as "this object is a *key*" or "this object is a *pencil*", with application of current midway during the stereotyped phrase. If the object was presented prior to stimulation, there would be no question of the availability of the name. This would tend to implicate articulation. It might also be of interest to see a description of patient errors, since aphasic patients are generally classified as much by misuse of language as by their linguistic poverty.

It should also be of interest to see the results of attentional tests during stimulation. Our finding that digit span was one of the more frequently impaired performances, and the common use of this test as an indication of attention span, lends support to objections based upon the role of distraction. Certainly, we know that anomia occurs normally in states of fatigue, inattention or distraction, and so this factor should be more carefully studied in future experiments.

In previous work, Dr. Ojemann has demonstrated that stimulation in subcortical white matter in right and left hemisphere produced similar effects. I am informed by him that such changes were more intensely anomic, without the paraphasic quality of intra-thalamic stimulation. This being the case, could not one suggest that thalamic stimulation produces only a less intense effect than subcortical stimulation? If so, then the latter would be expected to produce a stronger effect upon the target area in cortex, since the effect of intra-thalamic stimulation would be dissipated to some extent in the transmission to cortex.

Regarding the location of lesions in the pulvinar, and the sparing of the anterior-superior portion, I might say that I find it hard to believe that moving the lesion a few millimeters forward would have had so dramatically different an effect. Those of us who are engaged in the study of aphasia are just emerging from a long stagnant period of overly zealous cortical localization and I have a curious deja-vu about this starting all over again at the thalamic level. In this regard I am curious as to why Dr. Ojemann talks of "speech representation" in the thalamus. This has not yet been demonstrated to my satisfaction in his work and, besides, "representation" is a very provocative term.

## References

Brown, J., Riklan, M., Waltz, J., Jackson, S. and Cooper, I.: Preliminary studies of language and cognition following surgical lesions of the pulvinar in man (cryopulvinectomy). *Int. J. Neurol.* 8:276–299, 1971.

Bisiach, E.: Perceptual factors in the pathogenesis of anomia. *Cortex* 2:92–95, 1966.

## DISCUSSION

**Dr. Ojemann:** With regard to Dr. Brown's last questions, on the verbal memory test, all the trials that showed interference of recall had stimulation at current levels less than those interfering with object naming. It seems quite clear that the patient perceived to the point where he could name the object involved. So I think there is really no likelihood that perceptual disturbance plays a role in the verbal memory part of the task, as we presented it.

The problem of whether perceptual disturbance plays a role in the object naming part of it was a very real one for us. The way we tried to get around this in our particular task was to introduce the recall component of it.

What you find if you look at the performance on objects which cannot be named, as to how well can they be recalled, is that they can be recalled just as well, no better, no worse, than objects which are correctly named. So it seems that at least a proportion of these objects, which represent what we define as anomic responses are objects which are reasonably accurately perceived.

Another way we approached this was to use an auditory presentation rather than a visual one. We did that only in a very preliminary way and our initial impression of this data, at least, is the same in terms of the kinds of results one gets. So I doubt, although I'm not certain, that it is modality specific to visual input; at least as far as the object naming is concerned. The memory we just don't know. We haven't done the auditory input.

**Question from Floor:** I have two questions. One of them is, did you have an opportunity to study the polyglots, people who speak more than one language, and if you did, would that have any differential effect of pulvinar stimulation on the recall or the anomia of the first and subsequent languages?

And I had another question to Dr. Van Buren. Do you think that the phenomena described may be in some way related to the deficit of delayed alteration which has been observed in cats and monkeys from stimulation of the caudate nucleus?

**Dr. Ojemann:** To answer your question about polyglots, we had the chance to study one girl who was fluent principally in Dutch and slightly in English, and my recollection of that data was that there was no difference that we could demonstrate in the type of responses we got.

**Dr. Van Buren:** I really don't know, I was of course aware of the work on the frontal lobe by Mirsky and had done some of it. It struck me that this may be analagous to what we see in man. I think Larson did the nicest work on this. He has a lovely picture of a cat who had been trained to jump from one compartment to another over a type of tennis net by stimulating in the striatal area, I have forgotten exactly where it was, perhaps caudate, it was around the striatum; you could get the picture of the cat draped across the tennis net on his middle. It stopped him right between the two sides.

It strikes me that this probably is the same that has been reported in animals.

**Dr. Gilman:** I would like to ask Dr. Ojemann whether the parameters of stimulation he utilized might produce an augmenting response? If so, I wonder if that phenomenon might play a role in your observed speech abnormalities?

**Dr. Ojemann:** We have, on various occasions, looked for augmenting responses. I don't think we've seen them. I don't think we have looked on all the occasions when we've evoked anomic responses; perhaps some of them had them especially in the more anterior ventrolateral placements than we've had. We have looked for recruiting responses by changing our stimulus parameters. So far we haven't picked up those either. That would be a nice explanation for the improvement, for example.

**Question from Floor:** Dr. Ojemann, your results seem to concur with Dr. Cooper's. Most common postoperative changes seem to be decreased digit span and verbal memory and there was very little change in the comprehension of reading and conversation. Since the pulvinar is in close proximity with the hippocampus, and the mammillary bodies and fornix, is there any way of linking up a relationship between the pulvinar and memory rather than speech?

**Dr. Ojemann:** Well . . . if by that you mean is a current spread to these structures, I think the answer is clearly No. There are after all internal capsular structures at least between the pulvinar and hippocampus and you can pretty well tell when the current gets to the capsule you have a problem.

These patients don't show that response. If by that you mean anatomically, then I think the best guess is that it is the antero-temporal relationships of the pulvinar. I base that on Milner's data that not only are hippocampal complex structures impor-tant to verbal memory deficit, after at least temporal lobec-tomy, but also the lateral extent makes a difference. I think that is the most likely.

**Question from Floor:** Do you think that you're dealing with projection fibres at speech cortex? Do you think you are dea-ling with some intrinsic thalamic factor?

**Dr. Ojemann:** I have no way of answering that. Just as no one who stimulates or makes lesions in cortex can answer this since we have already seen today that pulvinar degener-ates with the cortical lesions in the speech area. I think the system works both ways, and I don't see how you can separate that.

**Dr. Fasano:** In two cases I did a simultaneous bilateral cryopulvinectomy. There are two types of patients included. The first are those with athetosis or dystonia and in these cases we have registered phonetic modification by means of electroacoustic recording. The record was carried out on a sonagraph, and the fine lines correspond to a normal vibra-tion of the vocal cords. So you can see letter A is preoperatively and letter B is postoperatively, while letter C is a normal voice. You can see in Slide B how it is changed to normal. The black lines improved and we have registered this kind of change in five cases. In one other we show very good modification of the phonetic responses. In other cases, you can see the Italian words, uno, dua, tres, quatro, and the best was where the vowels are present. It means that when you use the vocal cords more you have better response with cryopulvinectomy.

**Question from Floor:** What coordinates did you use for your lesions?

**Dr. Fasano:** We use another kind of lesion a bit different from the Cooper lesion. We place two lesions symmetrically. The first one 13.6 mm. behind the posterior commissure, that means 18 mm. from the medial commissural. The second lesion was 17 mm. laterally, 18 mm. behind the medial com-

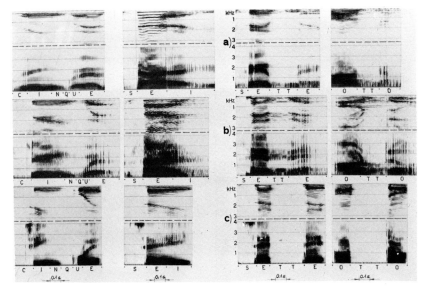

Figure 7–2. Phonetic modifications were evaluated by means of electroacoustic recording. In this slide we see three records:
A—Preoperative
B—Postoperative
C—Normal phonation
Recording was carried on with sonograph: Large track filter from 1 to 4 Khz (below) and narrow track with inverted frequency scale from 1 to 3 Khz (above).
Well defined lines correspond to a normal vibration of vocal cords.

missural line. In the first lesion the lesion was 2 mm. behind and above the posterior commissural line.

**Question from Floor:** May I ask whether these improvements in speech occurred with unilateral or did you need to have bilateral lesions?

**Dr. Fasano:** Phonetically, you mean?

**Question from Floor:** Yes.

**Dr. Fasano:** Unilateral.

**Question from Floor:** Does it make a difference whether it was left side or right side?

**Dr. Fasano:** Yes, rather left side.

**Question from Floor:** On the left side?

**Dr. Fasano:** Yes.

**Question from Floor:** And you mentioned that one patient had never spoken before.

**Dr. Fasano:** Yes. She spoke only a few words because she couldn't speak—not because she had not the facility to speak, you understand. It was because of the muscular spasm.

**Question from Floor:** So what you're suggesting is that there is no improvement of language but just in the capacity to make sounds?

**Dr. Fasano:** We have made very good improvement of swallowing in most cases. I think it is the same mechanism: the pseudobulbar syndrome in spastic children is improved.

**Question from Floor:** I'm sorry I'm confused on your lesion. The tip of your probe for one was lateral 13?

**Dr. Fasano:** Yes.

**Question from Floor:** Superior to and posterior to the posterior commissure, is that right?

**Dr. Fasano:** Yes. Two posterior and 4 above 13 mm.

**Question from Floor:** Lateral. And your second lesion was what?

**Dr. Fasano:** The second lesion was 17 mm.

**Question from Floor:** Lateral?

**Dr. Fasano:** And 18 mm. behind.

**Question from Floor:** 18 mm. behind the mid-commissure?

**Dr. Fasano:** Yes.

**Question from Floor:** So that would be about posterior 6 again? The same plane?

**Dr. Fasano:** 6.

**Question from Floor:** So posterior 6. And again your superior 4, and around, and that's the center of the lesion. How big do you think your lesion is?

**Dr. Fasano:** Well, I think the first lesion is mostly in the ventricular valley. We have no anatomical verification.

**Question from Floor:** Just in terms of the freezing period, what do you think the diameter is?

**Dr. Fasano:** 6 mm. each. Because we used minus 6°, not minus 120.

**Dr. Riklan:** Dr. Ojemann, were your results based only on stimulation studies?

**Dr. Ojemann:** Yes, these are stimulations. We've done acute studies on VL cases using the same memory test. If you use the Paterson type short term memory test, the one that I showed earlier, and do it on the second postoperative day, you find that people with left VL lesions do very much more poorly than preoperatively. People with right lesions do not do nearly so badly. In fact, most do the same as they did preoperatively. If you test object naming under these same conditions, you'll find that people with left VL lesions make far more errors. Nearly all of them showed some increase in object naming errors. The right showed a slight increase that was significant. There was also a significant difference between left and right. Both object naming and short term memory are disturbed by VL lesions. Of course, we have no experience with pulvinar lesions.

**Dr. Riklan:** Well, I think you have to add to what you said about those "that are disturbed by pulvinar lesions temporarily". There's much to say about this. Two days postoperatively you have an entirely different situation than even three days; certainly entirely different than seven days.

**Dr. Ojemann:** We purposely use the acute period because we want to maximize what we have seen.

**Dr. Riklan:** But then, when you use the acute period, you have no knowledge of whether you are measuring the specific effect of a VL lesion or the effects of a brain operation and all of its ramifications. That's one of the reasons we have tried to wait approximately a week following surgery, so that what might be called cerebral disorganizations, neural readjustment, the effects of edema, etc., all resolve to a degree and then we test. Any deficit one or two days postoperatively may be due to stimulation, I'm not sure. Maybe it is a function not of that specific structure, or those specific tissues, but it is a function of those tissues plus other facets of the surgical situation.

**Dr. Ojemann:** I would like to say that I do not entirely agree with that.

**Mrs. Jackson:** We undertook extensive speech and language evaluations with a patient before and after pulvinectomy. The initial speech evaluation of this patient (Mrs. D.M.) recorded her speech characteristics as overloud, explosive, bombastic and uncontrolled. The voice quality was overaspirate and hypernasal and there was a moderate dysarthria. Intelligibility was reduced more because of this uncontrolled repetitive delivery than the actual articulation.

Following the pulvinar lesion she acted and spoke much more calmly. Her voice quality remained overaspirate and hypernasal and there was still evidence of dysarthria, but her manner of delivery was what had changed so dramatically. She now had the ability to self-inhibit and her spontaneous speech as well as repetition took on a more "normal" rate and intensity, and everything she said was intelligible.

The pre- and postoperative evaluations of other patients who were noted to be dysarthric did not reveal any accoustical changes, but subjectively the patients reported that it "felt easier to talk". There were no patients in the study who were aphonic preoperatively who were able to produce voice postoperatively.

**Dr. Cooper:** Dr. Amin, Dr. Waltz and I followed the patient for a long time preop. I thought she was demented because she was shouting and screaming. With the pulvinar lesion, that change in her conversation took place and when I asked her if she was aware of it, she said yes that she was, and that previously she had simply been unable to control the bombastic repetitive speech.

**Dr. Brown:** I think we can confirm those observations. In some of our cases we did see speech improvement, not consistently, but occasionally, particularly in dysarthria. I remember one case in particular, with pseudo-bulbar speech, a very dramatic case. Severe pseudo-bulbar speech, speech with nasality, pressured speech in which we saw quite dramatic improvement following surgery.

**Mrs. Jackson:** I think Dr. Brown and I are talking about the same patient. This patient's speech was so bombastic that it was scarcely intelligible at times. And actually when we analyzed the speech after the surgery the qualities themselves were not that much different, it was the way she was able to inhibit her own speech so that it became more intelligible just in listening to it.

Most of the patients that we've done pre- and postop on tape have commented themselves that an improvement in speech has been a subjective thing. They say it feels easier to talk. The tape itself does not sound that much different pre- and postoperatively insofar as the dysarthria is concerned.

I don't recall a patient who had no voice who was able to get voice after surgery.

**Dr. Riklan:** In view of these findings, the question arises as to whether the change in the patient presented by Mrs. Jackson was an emotional-behavioral function or a speech function. It may have been an emotional change manifested by improved modulation in speech.

**Dr. Cooper:** I think that that's been generally the way I feel about it. And if, as Dr. Crighel suggested in his paper, the pulvinar modulates wide areas of the neocortex, raises or lowers the threshold somehow, perhaps in an opposite way than the head of the caudate, then I think we can begin to see a possibility of how all of these different functions can be modified under some circumstances without being able to have the specificity of rule of pulvinar.

# CHAPTER 8

# CLINICAL PHYSIOLOGY OF MOTOR CONTRIBUTIONS OF THE PULVINAR IN MAN: A STUDY OF CRYOPULVINECTOMY

I.S. Cooper, M.D., Ph.D., I. Amin, M.D.
R. Chandra, M.D. and J.M. Waltz, M.D.

THE PULVINAR is the most posterior and the largest of the thalamic nuclei. It merges rostrally with the nucleus lateralis posterior; the two regions share common cytoarchitechtural features and probably arise from a common anlage. It is of particular interest that its development is partially telencephalic in origin. In this regard its embryologic characteristics are shared with neostriatum (Rakic and Sidman, 1969). Phylogenetically, the pulvinar first appears in carnivores (Rioch, 1929); it becomes well defined in primates but only in man does the pulvinar attain massive size (Simma, 1957).

Anatomically the pulvinar seems dependent on the cerebral cortex. It is connected to the temporal (Siqueira, 1955; Van Buren and Yakovlev, 1959), parietal (Minkowski, 1923; Le Gros Clark and Boggen, 1935; Chow, 1950), and occipital cortex (Le Gros Clark, Boggen and Northfield, 1939) with rather dense afferent-efferent connection to the parietal cortex. It also receives afferent fibres from the pyriform cortex and amygdala (Papez, 1939). Recently, connection to the fastigial nuclei of the cerebellum (Snider and Sinis, 1971) has been demonstrated (Figure 1).

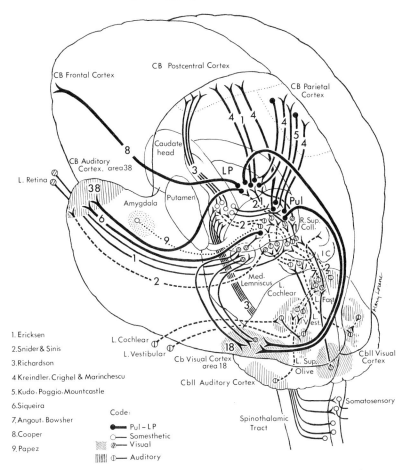

Figure 8–1. Diagramatic reconstruction of the LP-pulvinar complex connections. The principal connections ascribed to this complex as well as the original source of this information is indicated.

So little is known about the function of the pulvinar that Walker has referred to it as the terra incognita of the thalamus. Apart from the suggestion that it may be involved in the speech mechanism in man (Ojemann, Fedio and Van Buren, 1968; Penfield and Roberts, 1959; Van Buren, Yakovlev and Borke, 1969), the only evidence of other pulvinar function in humans comes from the work of Kudo *et al* (Kudo, Yoshii, Shimizu, Aikawa and Nakahama, 1966; Kudo, Yoshii, Shimizu,

Aikawa, Nishioka, and Nakahama, 1968; and Richardson (Richardson, 1967; Richardson and Zorub, 1970), indicating that the pulvinar plays a role in the process of pain appreciation. In cats the pulvinar has been shown to be a polysensory complex, in which neuronal pools respond to multiple sensory stimuli (Kreindler, Crighel and Marinchescu, 1968). Only recently has evidence been reported to indicate that pulvinar contributes to motor function (Cooper, Waltz, Amin and Fujita, 1971).

During the past months cryogenic lesions have been successfully made in pulvinar and lateralis posterior nuclei of the thalamus to alleviate abnormal tone, posture and pain sensation in 49 patients. Depth electrode and surface electrode recordings made during surgery aided in precise localization of the lesion and also in development of better understanding of anatomical and physiological pathways of these ill-understood subcortical nuclei. Preoperative and postoperative EEG recordings have also shown some significant changes.

The aim of this paper is an attempt to throw some light on the function of the pulvinar-lateralis-posterior complex in sensory-motor function in man through the analysis of 55 operations of cryopulvinectomy carried out in these 49 patients.

## MATERIAL AND METHODS

Fifty-five operations were performed on 49 patients. Twenty-one were males and 28 females. Most of the cases received two cryogenic lesions in the pulvinar but some had only one lesion and some had 3, including a lesion in LP. Nine patients had lesions placed in nucleus lateralis posterior, either alone or in combination with pulvinar lesions. Six cases were operated bilaterally. The principle indications for surgery were categorized in the following groups.

1. Dystonia
2. Athetosis
3. Spasticity
4. Torticollis
5. Intractable Pain

Following admission of the patient to the hospital, in addition to routine laboratory studies, all patients underwent clinical neurologic evaluation, EEG, language, speech, and psychological testing. Cinematographic records were made in each instance, including films during surgery when stimulation studies were carried out.

Operations were carried out using the same technique of cryothalamectomy described in earlier studies (Cooper, 1962). However, the target center used for the pulvinar lesion is placed at a point 17–19 mm. behind the midcommissural line on the lateral X-ray film and 3–4 mm. above it. This usually coincides with a point placed 4 mm. behind and 4 mm. above the posterior commissure. On the A.P. X-ray film the targets are taken 12 and 16 mm. from the midsagittal plane for medial and lateral pulvinar lesions respectively. For placement of a lesion in lateralis-posterior the target area lies 12 mm. behind the midcommissural line and 10 mm. above it on the lateral X-ray film. It is centered at 15 mm. from the midsagittal line on the A.P. X-ray film. (Figure 2).

Cryogenic lesions were created by a cryoprobe of 2.76 mm. in diameter. Within the target zone cannula tip temperature was lowered to minus 120° centigrade for 2 minutes in each lesion.

Electrophysiological studies during cryogenic surgery were done in 8 patients. Subdermal needle electrodes were placed in frontopolar, frontal, central, temporal, parietal and occipital areas on both sides on the basis of 10–20 international system. Surface EEG recording was bipolar in most instances. For monopolar EEG recordings, an indifferent electrode was placed on the cheek.

After the dura was incised and air ventriculography performed, an insulated stainless steel depth electrode with a spherical silver noninsulated tip was introduced stereotaxically toward the target. The depth recording was obtained between the tip of the depth electrode and a subdermal needle electrode on the surface of scalp near the burr hole. One millimeter above the tip of the electrode was a noninsulated silver ring. The two exposed silver contacts were employed

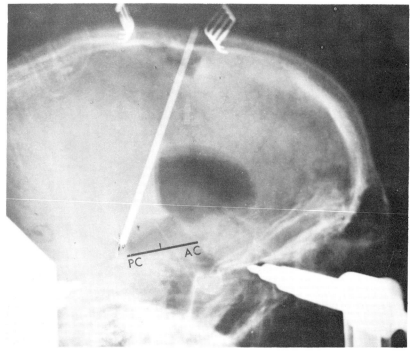

Figure 8–2. Roentgenographic landmarks used in placement of cryogenic probe into the pulvinar and LP.

for bipolar stimulation. A mechanical drive device holding the electrodes was placed in the stereotactic guide and was directed towards the pulvinar. The target point, the medial pulvinar, was 12 mm. lateral to midline and 4 mm. above and behind the posterior commissure. The spontaneous electrical activity at various depths was recorded as the depth electrode was driven to its target. Surface EEG and depth recording were simultaneously taken. Anteroposterior and lateral X-ray views were taken at intervals to identify the position of the depth electrode. Final placement of the tip of the depth electrode in pulvinar or lateralis posterior (LP) nucleus was always confirmed radiologically.

The surface EEG and depth electrode activities were recorded on a 16 channel polygraph EEG machine. The channels of EEG amplifier of interest were monitored by the oscil-

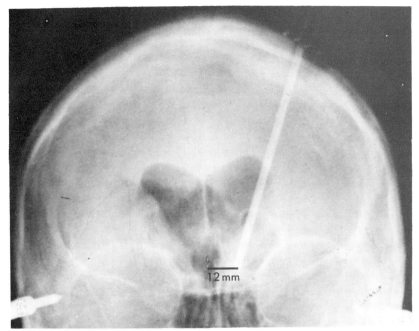

Figure 8–2B

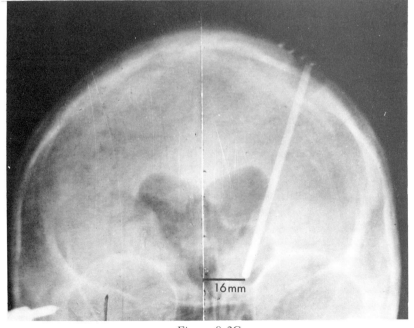

Figure 8–2C

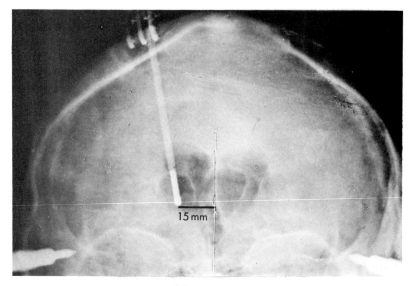

Figure 8–2D

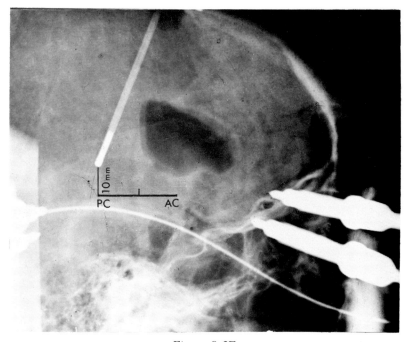

Figure 8–2E

loscope for latency period, amplitude and character of summated evoked responses. The 4 channel computer of average transients was used to examine EEG channels of interest for very small amplitude differences and sensitive evoked responses. The computer plotted out the summation by means of the x-y recorder. The stimulus was provided by the stimulater at voltages ranging from 3–20 volts of 0.5–1 m. sec. duration at a frequency varying from 1–20 cycles per second. Stimulation studies were performed on 8 pulvinar (4 left and 4 right) and 5 LP. (1 left and 4 right) nuclei.

Thirty patients who underwent cryogenic lesions in pulvinar and/or LP were subjected to preoperative and postoperative (within 7–30 days) surface EEG recordings.

## RESULTS

### A.   Electrophysiologic Observations

1.  Spontaneous electrical activity in cortical and subcortical structures: As the depth electrode was introduced stereotactically towards the thalamus, bursts of spontaneous activity in the cortex of 4–12 c/s, reduced in amplitude in white matter (Fig. 3a) and were replaced by characteristic large amplitude

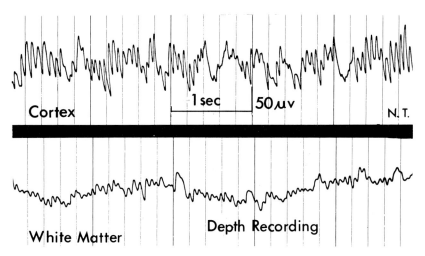

Figure 8–3a. Recording from cortex and from white matter as depth electrode advances to target area.

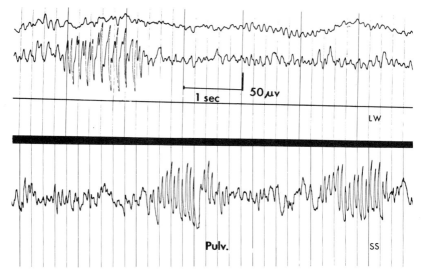

Figure 8–3b. Depth electrode within pulvinar demonstrating spontaneous spindling and rhythmic discharges.

rhythmic discharges when the electrode entered thalamic nuclei. This activity differed markedly from that recorded from white matter.

The pulvinar produced characteristic spontaneous spindling of 12–16 c/s and/or regular rhythmic activity at a frequency of 8–10 c/s. (Fig. 3b.) There was no characteristic trace obtained from lateralis-posterior nucleus except dense bursts of spontaneous activity ranging from 10–15 c/s. When the electrode approached the medial edge of the pulvinar the electrical activity was superimposed on pulsations transmitted from cisterna ambiens. This consistent phenomenon served as an additional localizing sign of electrode depth. (Fig. 4.)

2. Stimulation of Pulvinar: Rhythmic evoked potentials in the form of sharp and slow waves were obtained on surface EEG by stimulating the pulvinar at varying frequency and voltage with a pulse duration of 0.5–1 m. sec. The frequency and the amplitude of these evoked activities were related to the frequency and strength of the stimulating voltage. The EEG potentials appeared with the stimulus and disappeared

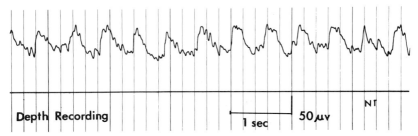

Figure 8–4. Transmission of CSF pulsation to the depth electrode as it approaches the edge of the pulvinar adjacent to cisterna ambiens. This serves as an additional localizing factor.

right after the stimulus was discontinued. (Fig. 5a.) There was no associated fatigue phenomenon and the EEG potentials appeared throughout the period of stimulation. The response was obtained principally in the ipsilateral temporal region but was also recorded from ipsilateral central and contralateral temporal regions. (Fig. 5b.) No motor or sensory phenomenon was clinically elicited during stimulation.

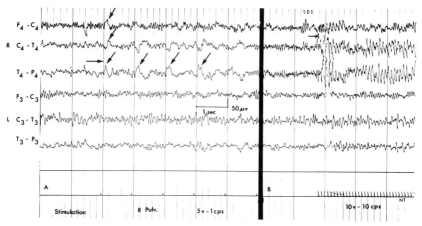

Figure 8–5a. Scalp electroencephlogram demonstrating evoked potentials resulting from stimulation within the right pulvinar. Stimulation at 5 volts, 1 c.p.s., produces evoked potentials in the right temporal region. 1 per second evoked potentials result in this instance.

Figure 8–5b. Stimulation of the same site within the right pulvinar at 10 c.p.s. resulted in evoked potentials, 10 per second, in the temporoparietal and central regions on the ipsilateral side.

However in two cases there was increase in muscular hyper-tonicity during pulvinar stimulation.

3. Stimulation of LP: EEG potentials were similar in appearance to those obtained when pulvinar was stimulated. The response was mainly recorded from ipsilateral fronto-central, but also from the temporal region. Contralaterally the responses appeared in centro-temporal areas. (Fig. 6.) Recording of superimposed single evoked potentials on an oscillograph demonstrated a latency period of 20 m. secs. and amplitude of 70 uv with a 5v, 5 c/s stimuli of 1 m. sec. pulse duration to the LP. Invariably, the stimulation of LP was associated with motor phenomenon, i.e., twitching of con-tralateral upper extremity with less frequent involvement of the lower extremity. This motor activity started distally in the hand or foot and spread to the more proximal parts of

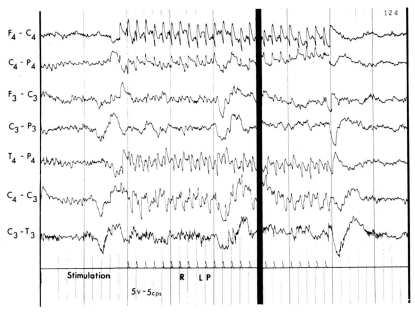

Figure 8–6. Stimulation in the right nucleus lateralis posterior at 5 volts/5 cycles per second, resulting in evoked potentials over fronto-central and temporal regions of the ipsilateral cerebral cortex. Stimulation could be carried out as long as 30 secs. without fatigue of the response. Onset and cessation of the evoked potential was virtually simultaneous with that of the stimulus.

the extremity. It continued for 1–2 seconds after the stimulus was discontinued.

4. Stimulation of VL: For control purposes identical stimulation of VL nucleus was carried out in certain cases in which it was the primary surgical target. EEG potentials with rhythmic slow wave discharges were obtained at a frequency of 10 c/s and a voltage of 10v in the ipsilateral central, and frontal as well as contralateral central and frontal region. However, fatigue on the contralateral side developed after 20 secs. and on the ipsilateral side after 30 secs. Continuing the stimulus did not produce an evoked cortical potential.

5. Effect of Freezing: There was no significant change in surface EEG during freezing or immediately after thawing of the LP or pulvinar lesion.

### Pre- and Postoperative EEG Studies

Thirty patients who underwent cryogenic lesions in pulvinar and/or LP were subjected to pre- and postoperative EEG recordings. The following lists the EEG observations made within 7–30 days following LP or pulvinar lesion infliction.

Following observations were made:

1. No change form preoperative status—11 cases.
2. Improved from the preoperative status—2 cases (In one case there was suppression of ipsilateral 3–4 c/s sharp waves). (Fig. 7).
3. Hemispherical slowing—4 cases.
4. Focal (Parieto-Temporal) slowing—7 cases.
5. Slow and sharp waves—3 cases.
6. Spikes and slow waves—3 cases.

Thus, 19 of 30 (63 percent) cases showed significant changes in EEG in the immediate postoperative period. Four of these developed one or more localized seizures in the postoperative period. Three of these four patients had suffered convulsive disorders prior to surgery. In these cases post ictal weakness (Todd's paralysis) developed. In 2 cases it was severe and took three weeks to resolve. In the other 2 cases the weakness was slight and full motor power was restored within 48 hours. In two of them, paroxysmal hemiballistic and

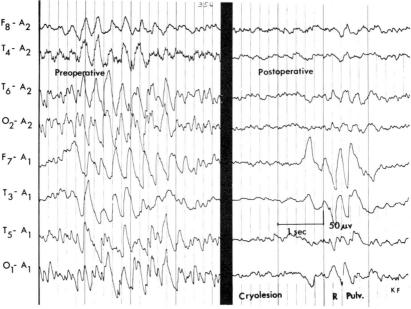

Figure 8–7. Disappearance of spontaneous 2–3 cycle activity noted in the preoperative electroencephlogram, following a cryogenic lesion in the right pulvinar. These bursts continued, however, in the contralateral hemisphere.

choreoathetotic movements of the corresponding upper limb preceded by several hours the epileptic attack.

In one of the two improved cases, cryopulvinectomy improved a psychomotor epilepsy refractory to temporal lobectomy and anti-convulsants. The patients had a few minor attacks in the immediate postoperative period and the post ictal paresis of contralateral side lasted for about 3 weeks. He was seizure free and his EEG tracings had improved at the end of six months. The other case of dystonia having bilateral sharp waves showed a suppression of these waves on the corresponding sides of the cryogenic lesion. She did not have any overt seizure either before or after surgery.

## B.   Clinical Observations

Lesions placed within the LP-pulvinar complex resulted in both motor and sensory responses which may be significant eventually in elucidating the function of this structure.

The motor responses were variable. This is undoubtedly due in part to the diversity of abnormal motor syndromes included in this series. A second factor rendering interpretation of the observed results difficult is the fact that most of the cases had undergone previous thalamic or cerebellar surgery. However, one fact does emerge from the data to be presented. That is, in a significant number of cases a clear cut modification of abnormal motor activity resulted from a pulvinar or lateralis-posterior lesion, which suggests that the LP-pulvinar complex may play a role in motor activity; a physiologic function not heretofore ascribed to this portion of the thalamus.

The sensory responses may be described as significant in both their positive and negative aspects. The positive observation is the fact that there may be an immediate striking relief of chronic pain, contralateral to a lesion within this thalamic complex, as previously reported by Richardson and Zorub, (1970), and Kudo *et al* (Kudo, Yoshii, Shimizu, Aikawa and Nakahama, 1966). The negative observation is the fact that such a lesion does not produce any observable objective change in perception of touch, pain, temperature, position, vibration, visual or auditory stimuli. Although sensory testing was clinically meticulous, it is certainly conceivable that sensory modifications not discernable by clinical testing do occur and will be defined physiologically by more sophisticated studies.

Evaluation included EEG, speech and psychological testing and pre- and postoperative motion pictures. A brief summary of the clinical observations follows:

*Dystonia Group*

Nineteen operations were performed on 16 patients with dystonia musculorum deformans or atypical unclassified dystonia. Twelve were females, four were males. All of these operations had been preceded by previous thalamic VL lesions with either incomplete relief or recurrence of the dystonic symptoms. (These patients were selected from a series of 300 dystonic patients who had undergone VL surgery. This series has been reported elsewhere).

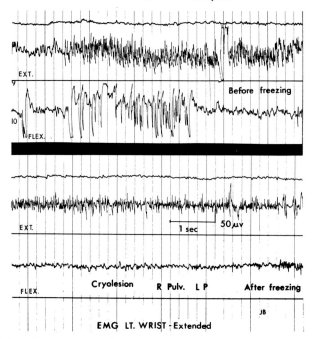

Figure 8–8. Electromyographic tracing from the left wrist flexors and extensor muscles before and after cryogenic lesions placed in the right pulvinar and nucleus lateralis posterior. Prior to freezing, extension of the wrist resulted in sumultaneous firing of flexor and extensor muscles. Following lesion placement wrist extension did not produce the flexor activity demonstrated preoperatively.

Of these cases operated in the current series ten demonstrated marked lessening of dystonic symptoms and six failed to show response to either pulvinar lesions or combined LP-pulvinar lesions. In this group, only pulvinar lesions were performed or combined LP-pulvinar lesions. (Fig. 8,9).

None of the cases showed worsening of dystonic symptoms following pulvinar lesions. One case showed an increase in dystonic symptoms subsequent to an LP lesion.

*Athetoid Group*

These were mostly patients with cerebral palsy, athetosis being the predominant feature of their clinical pictures. In most cases spasticity was present but this was not invariable.

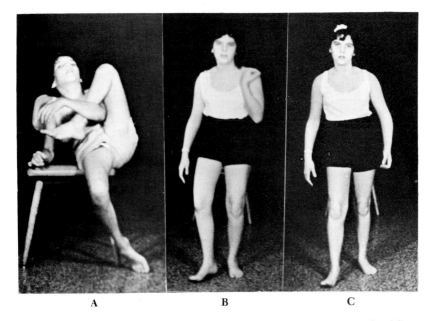

A           B           C

Figure 8–9a. A 14-year-old patient who had suffered severe disabling dystonia musculorum deformans involving all four extremities, the back, and the neck.

Figure 8–9b. This photograph demonstrates the patient following surgery in the left ventrolateralis nucleus, and left pulvinar. The cryothalamectomy in right ventrolateral nucleus has also been performed. Illustrated here is a residual marked rigidity of the left upper extremity which demonstrated severe spasticity and constant pain.

Figure 8–9c. The same patient following placement of a lesion in the right lateralis posterior nucleus. This relieved the severe spasm and pain present in the left upper extremity. Relief was instantaneous with placement of the lesion at the time of surgery. It is interesting to note that this patient has undergone bilateral VL surgery, surgery of the left pulvinar, and surgery of the right LP nucleus. No change in intelligence, emotional characteristics, speech or language has resulted from this combination of thalamic lesions in this particular patient.

Sixteen operations were performed on 15 patients. Seven were males and eight were females. Three of these patients had no previous surgery; while twelve had prior VL lesions, and two had also previously undergone cerebellar surgery.

Ten cases had significant useful relief of athetosis after surgery. Three had moderate improvement and three failed to improve. (Fig. 10 A, B.)

Thirteen of these procedures involved pulvinar lesions alone, while combined LP-pulvinar lesions were induced in the other.

It was difficult to assess voluntary motor power in this group of patients because most had little or no useful voluntary motion prior to surgery. However, there did appear to be a lessening of muscular power in 10 cases in this group, whereas motor power was unaffected in limbs in other groups which did not display weakness preoperatively.

*Spasticity Group*

This group includes patients whose main symptom was spasticity resulting either from a cerebro-vascular or traumatic cerebral lesion. Ten operations were performed; seven on males and three on females. Four of these patients had previously undergone ventrolateral nucleus surgery (usually for concomittant tremor). Two of the patients had cerebellar decortication and dentate nucleus ablation; two had LP surgery prior to or in addition to pulvinectomy.

Seven of these ten patients showed marked relief of spasticity (Fig. 11). None of them was rendered hypotonic. Three failed to improve.

*Miscellaneous Group of Involuntary Movement Disorders*

Seven operations were performed on five patients with miscellaneous diseases including torticollis and severe unclassifiable choreo-athetosis.

In one case of severe torticollis bilateral pulvinar lesions alleviated both the pain and abnormal posturing of the head and neck. In the remaining three operations no lasting effect was noted.

*Intractable Pain*

Thirteen cases operated in this series suffered from intractable pain. In three of these cases severe intractable pain was the principle indication for cryopulvinectomy. Two

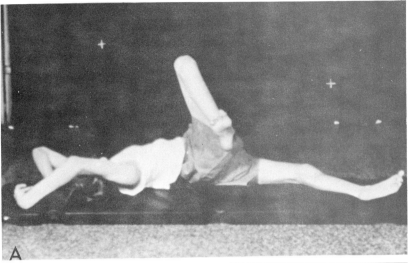

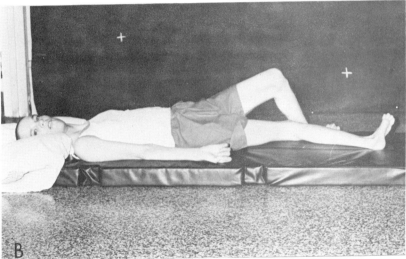

Figure 8–10a. A patient with severe spastic athetosis present throughout her lifetime.

Figure 8–10b. The same patient following left cryopulvinectomy. There was an obvious marked lessening of involuntary movements and spasticity contralateral to the lesion. Some degree of muscular weakness was noted following surgery. However, since there was no useful voluntary motor activity before the pulvinar lesion, the significance of this finding remains obscure.

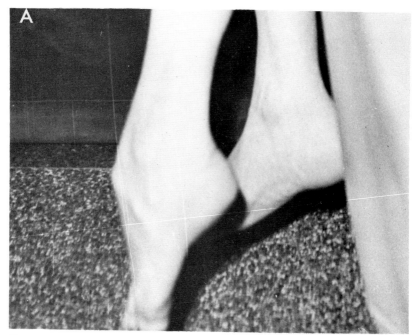

Figure 8–11a. A spastic deformity of the left foot of 2 years duration following a cerebrovascular accident. Surgery of the dentate nucleus of the cerebellum and VL nucleus of the thalamus had not affected this spastic deformity.

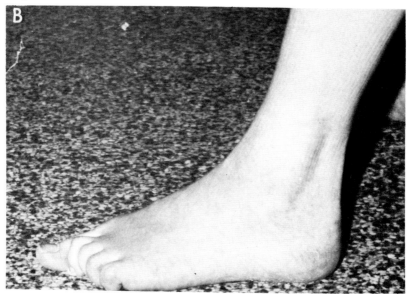

Figure 8–11b. Rehearsal of spasticity and deformity following cryopulvinectomy.

were cases of metastatic cancer, and one was due to long standing radiculitis which had not responded to medical therapy or cordotomy. All three were narcotic addicted. Pain relief was prompt and dramatic in all three patients.

Pain recurred shortly prior to death, 6 months post-operatively, in one patient with widespread metastatic cancer. It persisted up to the time of death (4 months) in a second patient with metastatic disease. The remaining patient is pain free 4 months following surgery without recourse to narcotics.

Ten other cases in which the primary indication for surgery was spasticity or involuntary movement disorder, severe intractable pain was also a principle complaint. In three cases the pain was burning hyperesthesia accompanying spastic hemiplegia. It was relieved in all three instances and has not recurred.

In the remaining seven cases the pain was due to severe joint deformity secondary to involuntary movement disorder. Six of the seven were relieved of pain. One of these recurred within two months.

Pain relief was specifically limited to pre-existent chronic pain. Perception of new or acute painful stimuli was not affected by LP or pulvinar lesions. No case in this series has been followed for more than 1 year.

## Bilateral Operations

Six patients underwent bilateral cryopulvinectomy. In two of them operations were performed at 10 days interval without ill effects. The other four cases had the second side operated upon after a 4 to 6 month interval. The bilateral procedures were well tolerated, without incident. Specifically, the dysphonic and/or dysphagic symptoms sometimes observed following bilateral ventrolateral nucleus lesions were not observed following bilateral LP-pulvinar lesions.

## Verification of Pulvinar Lesions

Three of our patients died at 3, 6, and 7 months following pulvinar surgery. Two died of cancer and the third died of subacute bacterial endocarditis superimposed on a mitral valve prosthesis. Post mortem studies showed the cryogenic lesions to be within the confines of the pulvinar (Fig. 12 A-B) in all three cases.

All lesions have also been charted for localization (Schaltenbrand and Bailey, 1959). In some cases the charting suggests the possible involvement of the posterior part of the body of the caudate nucleus within the edge of the lesion. However, no verification of this possibility is available at the present time.

*Speech and Language*

It is deemed important to note that neither speech nor language was impaired by either unilateral or bilateral LP or pulvinar lesions. An extensive study of speech, language and behavioral functions of the patients in this series has been carried out by Brown (Brown, Riklan, Waltz, Jackson and

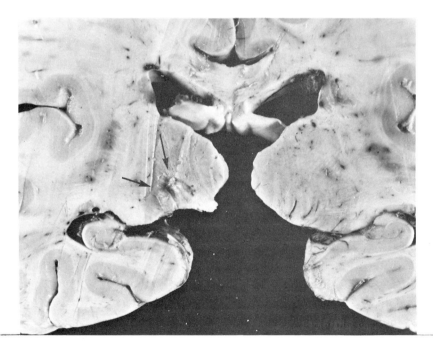

Figure 8–12a. Verification of the lateral cryogenic lesion in the pulvinar in a patient who died 6 months following cryopulvinectomy.

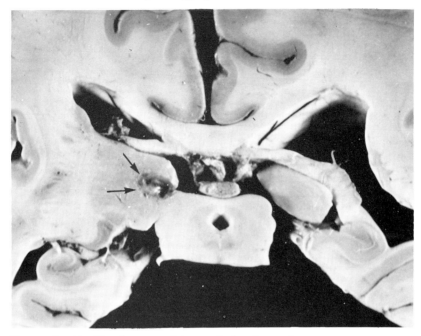

Figure 8–12b. Verification of the medial pulvinar lesion in a patient who died 6 months following cryopulvinectomy.

Cooper, 1971) and Riklan (Riklan, 1971), and will be the subject of separate reports.

*Side Effects*

1. *Temporary motor weakness* occurred in ten of our 55 cases. All of them recovered in 4–6 weeks postoperatively. The weakness appeared to affect the distal part of the limb rather than the proximal, was mild in eight cases, and marked in two cases.

2. *Sensory changes*—Three cases showed hypoesthesia on the side contralateral to the operated side. All recovered within the early postoperative period. In one case hypoesthesia of a mild degree (15% of normal) was detectable three months after surgery.

Except for the three patients mentioned above, no instance of objective sensory change, including touch, pain, temperature, two point discrimination, simultaneous stimulation of 2 loci, positive or vibration sensations have been impaired by the LP or pulvinar lesion.

3. *Behavioral changes*—One case showed mild agitated depression following pulvinar lesion which was easily controlled by medication. Two of our patients with compulsive aggressive tendencies appeared less so of these following pulvinar surgery. No other significant emotional or objective signs of intellectual or personality change have been observed.

4. *Seizures*—Four of our patients developed a focal seizure within the first week following the surgery. Three of these cases had a history of seizures before the pulvinar lesion was performed. One of these patients had a second seizure after hospital discharge but has now been seizure free for six months.

5. In one case of *severe bilateral spasticity*, in whom the right side had been relieved by left cryopulvinectomy, this spasticity recurred six months later, instantaneously, when contralateral surgery was performed for the left extremities.

There was no surgical operative mortality in this series of 55 operations.

### CASE REPORT

Mrs. D.M. was a 44-year-old right-handed female who was admitted to the Neurosurgical Department of St. Barnabas Hospital in November, 1970, because of left-sided hemiplegia, spastic in nature, accompanied with involuntary movements resulting from a cerebral vascular accident which she sustained in October, 1969.

Mrs. M. was noted to have had rheumatic fever in early childhood with rheumatic endocarditis. In 1963 she underwent a cardiovascular evaluation which was followed by open heart aortic valve replacement of that same year in December, 1963. She was doing well until October, 1969, when she had a sudden onset of severe pain localized in and behind the right eye. This was soon followed by loss of consciousness. She was hospitalized at that time. Clinical findings proved the presence of clouded consciousness, complete right third nerve palsy, left flaccid hemiplegia. Lumbar puncture performed at that time showed a clear CSF. During her stay in the hospital at that time, the patient showed progressive deterioration of her conscious level. Bilateral carotid arteriograms and right brachial arteriograms were done and were reported to be within normal, at that time.

The patient recovered consciousness but remained paralyzed on her left side. She was discharged from the hospital with left spastic hemiplegia and right third nerve palsy. She remained in that state until she was admitted to St. Barnabas Hospital in November, 1970.

Clinical neurological examination showed a conscious patient who was partially cooperative with an agitated depressive mood and occasional aggressive behavior. She was disoriented to time, place, and person, and she had an explosive type of speech. Cranial nerves showed complete right third nerve palsy. Both fundi were normal. There was a left UMN of left 7th nerve. The rest of the cranial nerves were intact. Motor system showed a posture of a left spastic hemiplegia. The left upper limb was adducted at the shoulder, internally rotated with a flexed hyperpronation at the elbow, flexion of the wrists with hyperextension of the fingers. The left lower limb was flexed, adducted and internally rotated at the hip, partially flexed at the knee. Ankle was plantar flexed and inverted. Tone was markedly increased, more in the flexor upper limbs and extensor of the lower limbs. Passive movements were markedly limited in all joints and persistence on trial would cause severe pain to the patient. Active movements were limited in the left side. Deep tendon jerks were markedly accentuated on the left side, up to 3+ and 1+ on the right. Left plantar showed positive Babinski signs. On the left side, the patient showed an arrythmic involuntary movement affecting the upper limb more than the lower limb. The patient could not walk or stand alone. She could be helped to stand up, but it was clear that her left foot would not touch the ground, because of marked spastic deformity.

Following admission to the hospital, routine laboratory

studies showed normal hemogram and normal urinalysis. Electrolytes were normal. Chest X-ray was normal. EEG was normal. Attempts to perform EMG and H-reflex were not successful because of restlessness of the patient.

*Course of Treatment*—On November 2, 1970 the patient underwent cerebellar surgery which consisted of open left posterior fossa approach, followed by decortication of Crus 1 and Crus 11 of the left cerebellar hemisphere. In addition to this, open resection of a core of the left cerebellar hemisphere including the left dentate nucleus was performed. The patient tolerated the procedure well. Postoperative period following cerebellar surgery showed no change in behavior, no change in speech, no change in cranial nerves. The changes were marked relaxation of tone, noted especially in the left upper limb. Passive movement was possible without pain. No change was seen in active movements and no change was noted in deep tendon jerks. Involuntary movement remained the same. The patient could stand up with support. However, the improvement following cerebellar surgery was short-lived. In two weeks time the patient's improvement completely disappeared. Her clinical picture in two weeks following surgery was exactly similar to her condition prior to surgery.

On November 17, 1970, the patient underwent a right cryothalamectomy under local anesthesia. The cryoprobe was advanced to a target situated 15 mm behind the posterior border of foramen monro, 2½ mm below the foramen-pineal line and at the distance, 9 mm lateral to the midline. Two cryo lesions were created by freezing down to −90 C for two minutes in each. This produced a large lesion in the ventrolateral nucleus.

Immediately following the right cryothalamectomy surgery, the patient showed complete disappearance of involuntary movements on the left side. Muscle tone was decreased but not completely relaxed. In two weeks, the patient was discharged from the hospital on a program of physical therapy. She continued to show some improvement in tone on the left side. Her condition on discharge showed cranial nerves to be the same as preoperative level. Speech was not changed.

One month later, examination revealed the patient to still demonstrate a spastic attitude of the left side but this was static and more marked distally, both in the left hand and left foot. Involuntary movements completely disappeared. Tone was moderately relaxed. Passive movements were easier to perform at all joints, except dorsiflexion of both left wrist aand left ankle. Limited active movements were demonstrated. Finger to nose test could be performed reasonably well. Sensation remained normal. The patient was able to stand up with the help of a brace.

Mrs. M. was readmitted to the Neurosurgical Department, St. Barnabas Hospital on May 30, 1971. She maintained the improvement she had gained from previous surgery. However, her clinical picture showed the following pertinent findings: (1) speech showed high pitch with an explosive character; (2) cranial nerves showed a right third nerve paresis; (3) motor system showed spastic posturing of the left hand and left foot, accentuated on attempts of active movement; (4) tone was spastic on the left side to a moderate degree; (5) deep tendon jerks were exaggerated with a positive Babinski on the left side; (6) sensation remained normal. The patient could stand up with the aid of a brace, but could not walk.

On June 1, 1971 the patient underwent a right cryopulvinectomy. Two lesions were placed in the medial pulvinar with freezing down to $-70C$ for two minutes for the first lesion and to $-120C$ for two minutes for the second lesion, which gave the patient an immediate reversal of the dystonic attitude of both left hand and left foot. Tone was markedly reduced and it was immediately apparent that the patient's speech improved. No complications were noted regarding level of consciousness, mentation, language. Field of vision was intact and no motor weakness, no sensory changes were noticed. Plantar reflex on left side remained extensor.

During her stay in the hospital, the patient maintained her improvement. In ten days time she began to walk with the help of a walker. The spastic deformity was totally reversed. She maintained an almost normal attitude of the left hand

and left foot, normal tone on the left side, improved motor function. Her speech lost its explosive nature and became normal.

On her last follow-up evaluation, (the patient was seen on October 20, 1971), the patient was alert, conscious and cooperative. Speech was normal. Cranial nerves still showed the right third nerve paresis. Motor system showed the patient to be able to stand straight up and to walk with some circumduction of the left lower limb. Attitude of the left hand and left foot was normal. Tone was relaxed on the left side. Babinski sign still existed on the left side. The patient demonstrated almost normal power on the left side, both upper and lower limbs. She was pain free. At that time, EEG tracing showed slow wave focus on the left frontal and temporal areas, but otherwise was normal.

Speech recording showed a definite improvement of speech. Speech characteristics on the initial evaluation were described as moderately impaired. Volume was over-loud and pitch was high, rising more with stress. Voice quality was over-aspirate, tremulous and hypernasal at times, markedly hyponasal and bombastic. Rate was uncontrolled and too fast with a staccato, explosive rhythm. Articulation was mildly dysarthric but generally intelligible. This is in contrast with her postoperative report which states that Mrs. M. exhibited a placidity in her speaking which had been almost nonexistent. Both volume and pitch were nearly normal. Rate was more appropriate and although her rhythm was slightly jerky there was very little of the former explosiveness. Voice quality remained over-aspirate and hyponasal with slight tremulousness and hypernasality. Articulation continued to be mildly dysarthric but intelligible. The impression of her overall speech changes suggest the possibility of psychological and/or neurological changes. Mrs. M. was now able to self inhibit her expressions.

On November 15, 1971, Mrs. M. became acutely ill, was admitted to the Passaic General Hospital suffering from hyper-pyrexia and she died on November 18, 1971, possible cause of death was a bacteria endocarditis of the aortic valve with multiple thrombo emboli. Post-mortem of her brain was performed at St. Barnabas Hospital and proved the presence of right cryothalamectomy lesion, right cryopulvinectomy lesions and left cerebellar decortication and dentatectomy, all to be anatomically correct. In addition, the lesion of her original midbrain embolic infarction that produced the left spastic hemiplegia was visualized.

## DISCUSSION

It has been our purpose to report these observations, which must be considered preliminary in nature, to illustrate the desirability of further multidisciplinary investigation of the LP-pulvinar complex in man. Because of its relatively recent phylogenetic development, evidence of a combined di-encephalic and telencephalic origin; its polysensory input; and widespread neocortical connections, it is an enigmatic structure of great interest and undoubtedly profound significance.

The characteristic spontaneous electrical activity from pulvinar gives a precise physiological localization while other subcortical nuclei viz. L.P., V.L., V.P.L., etc., only show non-specific bursts of electrical activity. Further advancement of depth electrode beyond the medial edge of pulvinar changes the electrical pattern to 2–3 c/s pulse wave indicating penetration into the quadrigeminal cistern or the cisterna ambiens. These observations were identical to those described by Albe-Fessard *et al.* (1961) and Guiot *et al.* (1962). Studies performed experimentally in cat by Richardson and Zorub (1970) found the pulvinar-activation to be independent of centre medianum, VPL and cortex in cats. Kreindler, Crighel and Marinchescu (1968) reported that the stimulation of pulvinar-LP complex in cats evoked responses in the homolateral as well as in the contralateral neocortical association and primary visual and auditory projection areas but never from posterior sigmoid gyri. They argued that the proper sensory interaction in pul-LP complex and the neocortical projection of the various points of these thalamic nuclei indicated the integrative role of this complex in transferring afferent impulses from one system to another and spreading them to large neocortical areas.

The appearance of evoked potentials on the cortex following stimulation of human pulvinar and LP nuclei in our study was very similar to that obtained by Kreindler *et al.* (1968) in cats. These electrophysiological studies in human patients strongly suggest widespread efferent projections from the pulvinar and LP nuclei of thalamus to the ipsilateral and contralateral neocortex, in keeping with previous anatomic investigations. (Simma, 1957; Siquiera, 1955). Stimulation of LP evoked responses more anteriorly on the neocortex than that of pulvinar.

Interestingly, surface EEG records taken during and immediately after cryogenic lesions in pulvinar and LP did not show any significant change. However, the surface EEG changes in 63 percent of the patients, in the immediate postoperative period, occurrence of epileptic attacks in 4 of them, paroxysmal choreoathetotic and hemiballistic movements in two of them preceding the frank seizures and subsequent clinical improvement with anti-convulsants point to the epileotogenic nature in some instances of the cryogenic lesion in pulvinar-LP complex at least in the immediate postoperative period.

We did not observe speech arrest during stimulation nor was there any speech deficit after placement of a cryogenic lesion in medial and lateral pulvinar or in lateralis posterior. This finding appears to be contrary to the observations of Van Buren *et al.* (1969) and Ojemann *et al.* (1968). Absence of speech arrest during stimulation in our cases may be due to the fact that in each of our cases medial pulvinar was stimulated whereas Ojemann (1968) indicated anterolateral pulvinar as the site of stimulation in his studies.

Stereotaxic lesions in the human pulvinar were first reported by Kudo *et al.* (1966) and by Richardson (1967) for the reduction of chronic pain. Both series showed the favorable effect of pulvinar lesion in the amelioration of pain appreciation without objective sensory deficit. No adequate explanation could be given based on the present known anatomical connections and physiological data of the pulvinar. The fact that a pulvinar lesion may lessen or abolish severe chronic pain without either interfering with perception of acute painful sensation or impairing the patient's affect is notable. The elaboration of the painful experience is one of the most complex of all clinical problems to decipher. The confirmation of the fact that LP-pulvinar may contribute to this experience initially seems only to cloud an already difficult physiologic problem.

However, since it is a fact, it will ultimately be useful in resolving the problem of pain mechanisms. To what degree pulvinar surgery can be useful for relief of intractable pain depends on further long-term clinical studies.

It is also apparent that mechanisms underlying various types of muscular hypertonus and hyperkinesis are complex and may be due to diverse co-existing mechanisms. The fact that stimulation of LP-pulvinar in the human may produce motor phenomena can presently be considered as an observation which merits investigation. The fact that placing stereotactic lesions of this structure may, at times, alone or in combination with other intracerebral lesions, lessen heightened motor tone has both physiologic and clinical implications. These cannot be assessed without considerable additional study.

Several observations concerning the effect of cryopulvinectomy on hypertonus and hyperkinesis merit mention. Our series demonstrated definite favorable effects in cases of spasticity and involuntary movements. Spasticity was markedly improved in the majority of cases operated for that symptom. The improvement seems independent of previous VL or cerebellar surgery performed prior to pulvinar lesions. Although the effect in some cases was striking, as exemplified in (Fig. 9, 10 and 11), it was not consistent. It appeared to be more marked on distal musculature than on proximal musculature. It appears to us to be strikingly different from the effect produced by a lesion placed in ventrolateral nucleus of thalamus.

The recently described connection between fastigial nucleus of the cerebellum and the pulvinar could explain the favorable effect of pulvinar lesion in muscle tone.

Delineation of the contribution of LP-pulvinar to motor function in an extremely varied clinical population will require extensive experience and meticulous evaluation. Likewise the clinical applicability of pulvinar and/or LP surgery to hyperkinetic states, alone or in combination with other lesions, cannot yet be adduced.

## CONCLUSIONS

The following preliminary conclusions are warranted on the basis of a detailed evaluation of the results of these operations.

1. It is possible to place large lesions stereotactically within the pulvinar and/or LP nucleus without any deleterious effect on voluntary movements, sensory, behavioral, or speech and language functions.

2. Although the effect of lesions within the LP-pulvinar complex varies depending upon the status of the sensory motor system of the individual patient, it is evident that these nuclei contribute to the control of muscle tone and motor function.

3. Partial ablation of the pulvinar may suppress or abolish intractable pain originating in the contralateral half of the body, without inflicting any sensory loss.

4. Although no objective evidence of intellectual or psychologic function has been adduced following cryopulvinectomy, the patients who are compulsive or extremely anxious appear less so following this procedure.

5. Evoked cortical potentials following pulvinar and LP stimulation by depth electrodes reveal a wide distribution of fibres from these nuclei to the ipsilateral and contralateral cerebral cortex.

6. The LP-pulvinar complex is a polysensory data processor, contributing to a wide range of somatosensory functions. Its role varies depending upon the functional condition of the individual brain.

## References

Albe-Fessard, 1961. Brown, J.W., Riklan, M., Waltz, J.M., Jackson, S., Cooper, I.S.: Preliminary Studies of Language and Cognition following Surgical Lesions of Pulvinar in man. *Intl. J. Neurol.* 8:276–290, 1972.

Chow, K.L.: A retrograde cell degeneration study of the cortical projection field of the pulvinar in the monkey. *J. Comp. Neurol.* 93:313–340, 1950.

Cooper, I.S.: Cryogenic Surgery of Basal Ganglia. *JAMA 181:*600–604, 1962.

Cooper, I.S., Waltz, J.M., Amin, I., Fujita. S.: Pulvinectomy: A preliminary report. *J. Amer. Ger. Soc. 19/6:*553–554, 1971.

* Kreindler, A., Crighel, E., Marinchescu, C.: Integrative activity of the Thalamic Pulvinar Lateralis Posterior Complex and Interrelations with the Neocortex, *Experimental Neurol.* 22:423–435, 1968.

Kudo, T., Yoshii, N., Shimizu, S., Aikawa, S., Nakehama, H.: Effects of stereotaxic thalamotomy to intractable pain and numbness. *Keio J. Med. 15/4:*191–194, 1966.

Kudo, T. and Yoshii, N.: Stereotaxic thalamotomy for pain relief. *Tohoku J. Exp. Medicine 96:*219–234, 1968.

Le Gros Clark, W.E. and Boggen, R.H.: The thalamic connections of the parietal and frontal lobes of the brain in the monkey. *Phil. Trans. R. Soc. B 224:*313–358, 1935.

Le Gros Clark, W.E., Boggen, R.H., Northfield, D.W.C.: The Cortical Projections of the Pulvinar in the Macaque Monkey. *Brain 60:* 126–142; 1939.

Minkowski, M.: Etude sur les connections anatomiques des surconvolutions Rolandique, parlietales et frontales. *Schweitzer Arch. Neurol. Psychiat. 12:*227–228, 1923.

Ojemann, G.A., Fedio, P., Van Buren, J.M.: Anomia from pulvinar and subcortical parietal stimulation. *Brain 91:*99–117, 1968.

Papez, J.W.: Connections of the Pulvinar. *Arch. Neurol. Psychiat. 41:*277–289, 1939.

Penfield, W. and Roberts, L.: *Speech and Brain Mechanisms* Princeton, Princeton University Press, 1959.

Rakic, P., and Sidman, R.: Telencephalic Origin of Pulvinar Neurons in Fetal Human Brain. *Z. Anat. Entwick, Cesc. 129:*52–82, 1969.

Richardson, D.E.: Thalamotomy for intractable pain. *Confinia Neurol. 29:*139–145, 1967.

Richardson, D.E. and Zorub, D.S.: Sensory Functions of the Pulvinar. *Confinia Neurol. 32:*165–173, 1970.

Riklan, M.: (1971, personal communication)

Rioch, E.M.: Study of Diencephalon of Carnivora. *J. Comp Neurol. 49:* 1–153, 1929.

Schaltenbrand, G., and Bailey, P.: *Introduction to Stereotaxis with an Atlas* of the *Human Brain Volume* II. Stuttgart, Georg Thieme Verlag; New York, Grune & Stratton, Inc., 1959.

Simma, K.: Der Thalamus de Menschenaffen, ein vergleichend-anatomische untersuchung. *Psyciat. et Neurol. 143:*145–175, 1957.

Siqueira, E.B.: Temporo-Pulvinar connections in the Rhesus monkey. *Arch. Neurol. 13:*321–330, 1958.

---

* Guiot *et al.,* 1962

Snider, R.S., and Sinis, S.: *Cerebellar influence on sensory relay nuclei of the thalamus.* Fulton Society, June 1971.

Van Buren, J.M., and Yakovlev, P.I.: Connections of the temporal lobe in man. *Acta Anat. 30:*1–50, 1959.

Van Buren, J.K., Yakovlev, P.I., Borke, R.C.: Alterations in speech and the pulvinar. *Brain 92:*255–284, 1969.

## DISCUSSION

**Voice:** I would like to ask whether Dr. Chandra thinks that the lesion in pulvinar is epileptogenic or whether the pass which would go through the vicinity of motor cortex would be the epileptogenic focus.

**Dr. Chandra:** We cannot hypothesize about this, but there is experimental evidence of epileptogenicity. I mean spikes were seen in the pulvinar and LP recordings, as well as from the surface and seizures were present.

**Dr. Cooper:** The course of the probe, is almost identical with that used in VL surgery and the incidence is less than 1% for a postoperative seizure in very large series of lesions so that was not a likely explanation.

**Dr. Gilman:** In producing your lesions of pulvinar, do you insert your cryogenic probe twice, or do you make only a single insertion as you generally do in producing VL lesions? If you make a double insertion, is it possible that you are producing greater damage to the cortex in the present series than in your previous work?

**Dr. Cooper:** I doubt that, because we have some cases in which we have operated six times. We have to work it out statistically but I don't think so. Due to our past experience it is not likely. Although we are saddened by the demise of three patients, we were able to get anatomic confirmation of our lesions, particularly since some of the motor responses had been originally unexpected and unexplained. So we are pleased to have been able to end with this demonstration that our charting and location is correct. I'm sure that's true of Dr. Richardson's series and Dr. Ojemann's. If there is no other remark on this paper, I will ask Dr. Gilman to begin to bring together some of the questions that have been raised in this long and interesting day.

# CHAPTER 9

# INVITED DISCUSSIONS

S. GILMAN, M.D., and L. POIRIER, M.D.

**D**r. Gilman: In opening the discussion of this most interesting symposium, I would like to begin by saying that Dr. Cooper has done a splendid job in organizing a very logical progression of papers, beginning with the embryology, proceeding through the anatomy to the electrophysiology, to the neurological, and then the behavioral, language, and clinical functions. I would like to discuss each of these very briefly; and discuss them by both making a few comments and also by perhaps interchanging ideas with the various individuals who have presented material today. And so, to begin with Dr. Rakic's most interesting presentation, he informed us about something that is quite new to me: that the pulvinar seems to be composed of two elements. One is some primordial cells that come from the ventricular wall and another group that seems to come from the GE, the ganglionic eminence. The ganglionic eminence in turn is responsible for the development of many other structures in the telencephalon in particular the basal ganglia, which gives us a link between the pulvinar and basal ganglia, a most interesting idea. It seems to me that histochemical studies should be directed along the lines of examining characteristics in common between pulvinar and caudate nucleus, putamen and outer globus pallidus. The medial globus pallidus, in contrast, seems to have a different origin. I think future experiments should be directed toward trying to understand which elements within the pulvinar have their origin in the ventricular lining cells as distinct from the GE cells. I would like to ask Dr. Rakic if he has any speculation about this and, secondly, I wonder what is the ultimate origin of the GE cells.

**Dr. Rakic:** Well, I think you outlined rather well the direction that research in this area should take. The problem is that the precise tracing of the cells which originated in the ganglionic eminence would be possible only after thymidine-$H^3$ administration *in vivo* and subsequent preparation of brain tissue for autoradiography, an approach which cannot be applied to humans. Aware of that, we began experiments with thymidine-$H^3$ injections in a series of pregnant rhesus monkeys. Our rationale was that the pulvinar, though not developed as much in the monkey as in man, has evolved more than in any subprimate species. At present we can only speculate on the basis of other examples where neural structures were found to have dual origin. For instance, in the cerebellum, cells of early origin become confronted subsequently with a wave of late-forming cells. In such cases, as pointed out in my presentation (Rakic, this symposium), the first elements to develop are "large cells", their size actually being not as important as the fact that these cells usually have long axons and therefore make a basic framework of long interconnections between distant regions. M. Jacobson has argued that these early-forming large cells also may be genetically much more rigid, and morphologically more stereotyped. Later-forming cells are usually smaller and more versatile; most of them differentiate into interneurons scattered among the larger neurons. One may speculate that the pulvinar follows a similar history. Of course, this remains just a speculation since there are also exceptions to this rule. The other question?

**Dr. Gilman:** Can you trace the origin of the GE?

**Dr. Rakic:** The ganglionic eminence develops initially as an enlargement or swelling (hence the name "eminence") that projects into the lateral ventricle at the base of the telencephalon. Some of the pioneer cells that originate in the ventricular zone secondarily move out and form a new layer, the subventricular zone, in which they continue to proliferate. It seems reasonable to classify ganglionic eminence as an especially enlarged subventricular zone.

**Dr. Gilman:** I would like to discuss next the very interesting anatomical points raised in the presentations of Dr. Siqueira and Dr. Van Buren. A problem arises when one attempts to interrelate anatomical with electrophysiological findings. The obvious discrepancy is that one has electrophysiological communication between structures that have no demonstrable anatomical connections, as shown by the techniques utilized in the studies of Γ. Siqueira and Dr. Van Buren. However, there are problems in these kinds of studies. If transsynaptic degeneration does not result from a lesion, one may not be able to demonstrate a multisynaptic pathway by the technique of lesioning and conventional staining. The techniques that Drs. Siqueira and Van Buren have utilized have been fiber degeneration or Marquis and Nauta stains, as well as gliosis and neuronal changes after a lesion.

In Dr. Van Buren's studies the lesions were made in humans and anatomical studies were made a long period of time after the lesion had been placed. It is interesting to note that, for a long time an eminent neuroanatomist, Dr. Malcolm Carpenter, denied that there were connections between the substantia nigra and the basal ganglia, particularly the caudate and the putamen. However, he has recently utilized a new technique, the Whitaanen technique, which can trace very finely myelinated fibers, and he has now confirmed what the fluorescence microscopists and electrophysiologists had already demonstrated: that is, that there are important connections between substantia nigra and the striatum, and these connections are vitally important in Parkinson's disease. The point of this comment, though, is that one must not restrict one's thinking anatomically to just monosynaptic connections of large diameter myelinated fibers. One must think also about the small diameter fibers and multisynaptic connections, in thinking about the connections of a structure like the pulvinar.

It is conceivable that some of the connections that have been described classically may be only a small fraction of the important connections of the structure. Dr. Frigyesi's demonstration of a neuron in pulvinar, responsive to stimulation in caudate nucleus, medial thalamus and probably putamen, is clear evidence that there are functional connections between pulvinar and other portions of the deeper grey

masses in the brain. In connection with Dr. Frigyesi's demonstration, I would like to know the latency of the onset of
your effect.

**Dr. Frigyesi:** The latencies in pulvinar to all modes of stimulation in the responsive neurons were similar to the latencies
we have observed in the nucleus ventralis lateralis under
similar conditions. In the entopeduncular nucleus, the onset
of the EPSP was definitely rising by about 4 milliseconds,
by 3 or 4 milliseconds, which is approximately 1 millisecond
more than what we had seen in VL. In the second electrophysiological slide which I have shown, the onset of the
IPSP in the putamen neuron during caudate stimulation
was 12 milliseconds.

**Dr. Gilman:** A series of well placed lesions could help
to solve the problems of the route into the pulvinar from
your central electrical stimulation sites. The long latency
responses you showed and the neuroanatomical problems we
have seen leave it up to the electrophysiologist to work out
the pathway. Dr. Frigyesi and Dr. Cooper may recall a similar
problem we had with respect to the vestibular system, the
argument being that there are no anatomically demonstrable
projections rostral to the posterior commissure, which is man-
ifestly absurd. One needs careful lesions in an electrophysiological setting to unravel the anatomical connections, and then analyze their function.

This leads us into discussions of the effects of stimulation
within the pulvinar and in this context it is appropriate to
think about the very interesting data of Dr. Crighel, and also
of Dr. Ojemann. First, it is obvious that Dr. Ojemann has
been controlling very carefully his parameters of stimulation.
It seems clear that his stimulating current is not spreading
across into the internal capsule because he has not observed
motor responses during stimulation. It also seems clear that
many of the projections he is activating by stimulation emerge
from the pulvinar and proceed to temporal lobe, possibly
to occipital lobe, and also possibly to the parietal-occipital
interface. Accordingly, I would like to suggest an explanation
for his results that may best be expressed succinctly as a
*busy signal* effect. There is a well-known study in experi-

mental psychology in which a subject is asked to speak extemporaneously while he is being fed back through earphones the words he has just produced, with a delay of some milliseconds. The experiment is accomplished with a tape recorder and a simple timing circuit. The effect of the feed-back speech is to cause the subject to speak jargon. Viewed from another angle, this experiment indicates that the nervous system speech apparatus breaks down when it is flooded with a particular kind of auditory input. I wonder whether Dr. Ojemann's studies provide a similar type of "stress" on the mechanisms of visual cognition and speech. Dr. Ojemann stimulates within the thalamus and produces a disorder in the patient's capacity to recognize a symbol. This is all visual, as Dr. Brown correctly pointed out earlier. In his incapacity to recognize a symbol he produces a wrong word or develops what Dr. Ojemann terms a disorder of recognition. I wonder whether it could be that there is a "busy signal" on the line; in other words, your electrical stimulation has so flooded the nervous system with activity that the appropriate areas of cortex are incapable of responding to other stimuli. I should hasten to add that this is a simplistic and perhaps overly naive explanation, but one wishes to have some meaningful frame of reference for understanding the effects you observe with electrical stimulation when Dr. Riklan and Dr. Brown have found that quite large lesions in pulvinar do not disturb the speech mechanism. I shall be interested in your reflections about this problem, Dr. Ojemann.

**Dr. Ojemann:** Well, I think the stimulation is analogous to putting in a busy signal. This is probably a reasonable parallel. This is true whether it is cortical stimulation or whether it is subcortical. The problem one runs into, if you are going to envision this, however, as a disruption of a general organized system in the left brain, is that there are differences depending on whether you put the stimulus in the parietal white matter, pulvinar ventrolateral thalamus, or in the temporal parietal, all of which we have published. And the effect of this on speech or verbal memory on both tests are somewhat different. The differences are somewhat subtle but they are very real. So it isn't just a matter of putting noise in the line, it depends on exactly where you put the noise in terms of the kinds of results you get. I think beyond that, that the difference from area to area seems to provide the best data to suggest the effects have anatomic specificity, in addition to the obvious fact that in VL thalamus, we have good indication of points that do not give us disturbance of speech object naming functions and points which do.

**Dr. Riklan:** Another question which arises in this context is the differentiation between speech and language and this is something we could discuss for a long time. The changes you have reported were in language. That is the use and understanding of a symbol of an object or a concept. But that is not the only possibility here. I think what also might be happening is that the motor aspect of the speech system may be involved. As I recall, in Guiot *et al.*\* paper in 1961, an arrest in speech occurred following VL stimulation, the implication being that what was happening was that speech was being arrested rather than a loss of the language symbol of the object. I don't know whether we can resolve this question. It might be a combination of the two.

**Dr. Ojemann:** I think that distinction is one we can readily resolve. Anomic patients have language and speech functions, in that they can say things—fairly complicated things—like: "I don't know what that is." So it isn't a matter of the motor speech function not being there. It is very clear—there is such a thing as an arrest response. The patient is unable to respond, whether this interferes with consciousness or output, or what have you. And that's different from the anomic response when the patient demonstrates he can respond in terms of a motor output system, but he can't identify the object. It seems much more likely that the anomic response represents a language disturbance, and was associated with prolonged aphasia: aphasia that persisted for the survival of these patients. And we obviously do have a problem with most of the lesion data that has been presented here today, in that the majority of the lesions for which we have anatomy

\* Guiot, G., Hertzog, G., Rondot, T., Molina, P. Arrest or acceleration of speech evoked by thalamic stimulations in the course of stereotaxic procedures for Parkinsonism. *Brain, 84,* 363–379, 1961.

verified, in fact, do not impinge on that part of the pulvinar where our electrodes have been located. They have been distances away, distances getting close to a centimeter; which is a big measure in the thalamus.

And I think that this issue simply remains open. I don't know whether the lesions which turn out anatomically to be lateralis posterior of the dominant side are going to show transient, like VL, or more persisting speech or language disturbance.

**Dr. Gilman:** To take up next Dr. Crighel's presentation, he showed a post-tetanic enhancement of flash-evoked response by stimulating within the pulvinar and he found both homolateral and crossed effects. I find it difficult to accept these findings as presented because of the possibility that a spread of stimulating current may cross the midline.

Accordingly I would like to ask him whether he has attempted the same kind of experiment with a sagittal section of the tectum to determine whether he is activating a system which goes from pulvinar down to tectum and then across to the other side and back up to cortex again, or a system that goes from pulvinar to occipital cortex, then across the posterior corpus callosum to the opposite cortex?

**Dr. Crighel:** I cannot believe that it was a spread of the stimulating current because:

(a) We did not find a direct relation between the intensity and duration of the stimulating current and the contralateral effect, but the relation, as it was shown, was in some instances inverse.

(b) In previous investigations we showed that the LP stimulation elicited responses in the contralateral LP with shorter latencies than the responses from the contralateral neocortex and these responses remained unchanged after the disappearance of the responses in the homolateral neocortex following a spreading depression elicited by KCl.

We have not made a sagittal section of the tectum but we performed experiments in animals with pretectal section, with the same results. Therefore we consider that the contralateral effect is mediated, in cat, by a route passing through massa intermedia, from the pul-LP complex to the contralateral pul-LP and then to the opposite neocortex.

**Dr. Gilman:** Thank you. With respect then to Dr. Trachtenberg's presentation, which also bears upon the question of stimulation effects in pulvinar, I would side with Dr. Frigyesi in criticizing the thesis that Andersen has put forward. I don't believe that it is tenable in the light of evidence that has been generated from a number of different laboratories, particularly that of Dr. Purpura. Nevertheless, it certainly appears that stimulation within the pulvinar, provided one uses the proper parameters, is capable of producing rhythmical discharges from large areas of the cerebral cortex. The work of Dr. Chandra and Dr. Cooper, presented today, supports this idea. I wonder if Dr. Trachtenberg would tell us where he thinks the pathway might be located which produces the kind of cortical activation that he demonstrated?

**Dr. Trachtenberg:** As we all know, there are obvious pathways running from the pulvinar to much of the temporal-parietal and occipital cortices and return pathways from these cortices to the pulvinar. The first and obvious suggestion, of course, is that these pathways are mediating the response that we have seen. While we are on pathways, I don't know the situation in the human but in lower forms there is a pathway from the dorsal thalamus ventrally via the postoptic commissure to the contralateral dorsal thalamus. This might be mediating Dr. Crighel's responses.

**Dr. Gilman:** That's a nice idea. Just to return for a moment to your findings upon stimulation in the pulvinar, if I understood it correctly, when you stimulated in the left pulvinar, you would get a deviation of the right eye to the right. What movement would the left eye make? I believe your diagrams indicated a vertical movement.

**Dr. Trachtenberg:** The left eye deviation varied as a function of the stimulus locus. So that in some cases it went up. In some cases it went down, but the changes were really very small. We are talking about 1½ degrees or so as opposed to something like 4 or 5 degrees deviation in the right eye. So these changes are really quite small. The most prominent deviation is actually in the vertical plane.

**Dr. Gilman:** I believe your observations raise the possibility that you are stimulating some pathway that dips down into the tectum and possibly even descends as low as the pons. The reason for this comment is that, in a sense, your stimulus produces a skew deviation. The site in the nervous system thought to be responsible for skew deviation is the cerebellum and its brainstem connections, particularly the pons.

**Dr. Trachtenberg:** Examination of the brain of one monkey which had a section of the corpus callosum and was stained by a variant of the Nauta technique revealed fibers leaving the internal capsule, coursing through the dorso-caudal aspect of the ventral posterolateral nucleus and the oral pulvinar to terminate in the pontine nuclei and parts of the nucleus reticularis pontis.

**Dr. Gilman:** The electro-oculograms you showed were very interesting. Initially, as I recall, you found saccadic movements when a patient was asked to read, and then, as the patient continued to read, the eye movements became continuous. This observation is striking in the light of the concept elaborated by Daroff and Hoyt (*The Control of Eye Movements,* Academic Press, Inc., New York, 1971, pp. 175–235). There are two separate systems for eye movements. One is a system subserving saccadic eye movements, utilized during "voluntary gaze", mediated from the frontal cortex to the pontine paramedian reticular formation. The second system, which subserves pursuit movements, utilizes continuous ocular movements which are initiated in the occipital-parietal cortex and are mediated also by pontine paramedian reticular formation. I wonder if you were demonstrating saccadic movements during the initial portion of the task and pursuit movements later. I also wonder whether stimulation of pulvinar produced only pursuit movements.

**Dr. Trachtenberg:** First of all, the electrical stimulation parameters were such that the current density was extremely low. It was something of the order of 1/10th to 1/100th of that usually used in animal experiments or of that discussed today. On the other hand, the duration over which stimulus had to be applied to get a response usually was quite long. Frequency was 60 per second. The movements were, as you saw, initially fast followed by a rather slower phase. All in all we should call them pursuit type movements rather than saccadic movements.

This is what one would expect from stimulation of the pulvinar considering that it has a profound connection with areas 18 and 19, which should be responsible for pursuit type movements. If we had gotten saccadic movements I would have been more surprised.

**Dr. Gilman:** I completely agree and your observations are very interesting. In attempting to discuss Dr. Richardson's presentation, I find myself at a loss on several counts. First, I believe he is using a stimulus of such great intensity that he is activating a large number of different kinds of fibers, nociceptive, muscle, proprioceptive, joint proprioceptive, etc. Then he found that he would lose his response in pulvinar with combined lesions of dorsal columns and mesencephalic reticular formation. However, an early component of the response was preserved. I find it very difficult to understand what is happening in these experiments, and wonder if he has tried the control of completely sectioning the cord in these preparations, just to make sure that the early component is not an artifact of some sort.

Dr. Richardson's presentation carried us into the question of pain and the effect of pulvinar lesions in relieving pain. I think this is a very exciting new concept, if it proves to be correct. I believe that we should be very cautious in drawing any conclusions at this early stage in the clinical investigation of pulvinar lesions on pain, since we must regard the therapeutic effects as unproved at this point. Furthermore, we have little information on the mechanism involved, though I doubt very seriously that it could involve interruption of classical "pain pathways". The traditionally accepted pathway involves the spinothalamic tract at a low level and the reticular formation and related thalamic nuclei at a high level, and the pulvinar has not previously been considered to be one of those pathways. Furthermore, as we are all aware, there are complex psychological factors involved in the detection of pain and in the emotional response to it, as Wall and Melzack have pointed out in their writings. We are confronted with a most interesting situation, in which patients with pulvinar lesions have no loss of primary sensation and yet they don't perceive deep pain, nor are they bothered by applied deeply painful stimuli.

Dr. Richardson took care to say that his patients did not have the abnormalities classical of patients with frontal lobotomy. I believe that Drs. Riklan, Waltz, and Cooper have made similar observations in patients subjected to pulvinar lesions in this hospital. Dr. Cooper has kindly allowed me to examine some of these patients, and I agree that no loss of sensation can be demonstrated by classical neurological examination. However, it is possible that the patients have a defect too subtle for our testing.

There may be, in fact, an emotional abnormality which we simply do not have the tools to test for. Until we have the appropriate tests I think the question must remain open. However, I doubt very much that the pulvinar can be viewed as any sort of "pain termination center"; my guess is that the lesions alter the patients' emotional reaction to pain.

This leads into another area that I would just like to comment upon briefly, which is Dr. Riklan's provocative statement that a variety of thalamic lesions in dystonic patients do not seem to remove any psychological function that we can measure. I think these lesions must impair the function of the nervous system in some way, but I fear our measuring tools may be simply inadequate to detect the abnormality. In recalling Lashley's experiments of many years ago, we may have a comparable situation. He ablated one part of the brain after another and yet rats could retain the capacity to follow a maze, so that he finally concluded that memory has no focal localization. However, more recent clinical and experimental observations indicate that hippocampus and medial thalamus are important foci for certain types of memory. Thus, we must ask ourselves whether our testing devices are adequate to provide an answer to our question.

**Dr. Riklan:** You may be correct, but I think we are talking from a different perspective. Theoretically each neuron in the brain has a role, a function. If one neuron is destroyed then theoretically a function may be taken away. But as we look and examine people, I don't know whether it is simply a matter of tools. I think that perhaps a function may be lost but it may be a function somehow quite adequately assumed by other neural means. Now dystonic patients who have five or six lesions may lose something that better tools could assess. But in final reduction of such a statement that each neuron has a function, I think it's impossible clinically to measure possible losses.

**Dr. Gilman:** Well, when one places a lesion of about 3mm diameter in a structure obviously highly evolved such as the pulvinar, and detects no clinical abnormality, I submit that it is our detection device that is faulty, and not that the brain doesn't need the pulvinar. I would just like to make one further comment related to the very interesting motor effects that, in fact, result from lesions of the pulvinar. We don't understand the mechanism by which they relieve spasticity or dystonia, and we need considerably greater experience before we can conclude that they produce reliable, beneficial effects in patients. In my limited experience of examining some of Dr. Cooper's patients, the effects of pulvinar lesions seem to vary considerably from one patient to the next. In one patient a pulvinar lesion added to a VL lesion will produce a remarkable amelioration of a dystonic posture and in another patient it seems to do very little. I don't think we even understand why VL lesions are beneficial in relieving rigidity. However, I would like to make a proposal along these lines, which is that lesions in ventrolateral nucleus interrupt a circuit that is important in the facilitation of the spinal motor neurons by way of the gamma motoneuron system.

I would now like to show a few slides to document this statement. The slides illustrate results from a series of experiments that my colleagues, Drs. Lieberman and Copack, and I have carried out recently. We have placed a probe in the ventrolateral nucleus of the thalamus and have progressively cooled the VL nucleus while measuring the responses to stretch of muscle spindle primaries located in the gastrocnemius muscle of lightly anesthetized, otherwise intact cats. We have found consistently that a freezing lesion in the VL nucleus produced by lowering the probe tip temperature to $-20°$ C to $-40°$ C results in a significant depression of the responses to stretch of the spindle primaries. The design of these experiments permits us to conclude that the depression of the responses to stretch results from a decrease of tonic gamma (fusimotor) neuron activity. We have conducted similar experiments in which we place our probe in the pulvinar and freeze progressively while measuring responses of spindle afferents in the same way we did during ventrolateral nucleus freezing. The results were very clearcut: despite cooling to $-60°$ C, producing large lesions, we found no significant depression of spindle responses.

Consequently, we feel confident that the VL nucleus of the thalamus is an important relay station in the control of fusimotor activity, but the pulvinar is not. We have other evidence bearing on this point. For the past several years, my colleagues and I have studied the effects of lesions in cerebellum, precentral cortex, and medullary pyramidal tracts on the responses to stretch of muscle spindle afferents. Much of this work has been done in the macaque monkey and has been published over the past several years. Our findings can be summarized briefly by stating that, in general, hypotonia of the limbs resulting from these lesions correlates very well with a depression of spindle afferent responses to muscle stretch owing to a decrease of fusimotor activity. We have therefore developed the concept that there exists an important series of relays in the central nervous system that are vital to the maintenance of tonic fusimotor activity. These relays comprise a cerebello-thalamo-cortico-spinal system "wired" into the fusimotor neuron. The ventrolateral nucleus of the thalamus appears to be part of this system but the pulvinar does not. Accordingly, perhaps VL nucleus lesions are effective in relieving rigidity by depressing fusimotor efferent discharge, which, in turn, would result in a depression of tonic alpha discharge to muscles. Since pulvinar lesions do not affect spindle responses, perhaps these lesions affect alpha motoneuron firing in some manner independent of the fusimotor neuron. This is a possibility that Dr. Cooper suggested about nine months ago. Thank you very much.

**Dr. Cooper:** Thank you Dr. Gilman—that has been an excellent exposition of the problems that have been raised. I would like to take one minute to discuss your discussion as related to the motor system. About four or five years ago I gave a paper at the Academy of Neurology in which I suggested that there was an effect on the gamma motor system following a VL lesion. My own hypothesis at the moment is that there is an obvious difference between the unpredictable effect of the pulvinar lesion on the motor function and the quite predictable effect in VL.

On the other hand, thousands of VL lesions have been placed in humans and the indications are defined. In pulvinar, as you know, we have done a heterogenous group of cases of almost indefinable description, and some effects have been very marked and some have been absolutely nil. I feel and I was quite struck by the work of Dr. Crighel, in the cat, that there is an augmentation of cortical response across the board from pulvinar, and that will depend upon the state of the patient, his age and his disease, and everything that has been going on in his lifetime. Any augmentation or contribution to motor function probably takes place by way of the cortex and then down.

That may not be so but certainly I agree that there is a difference and it is not only on spindle, but whatever effect we have seen here takes place.

**Dr. Ojemann:** I wonder if I could comment briefly on Dr. Gilman's last presentation. Those of us who work with Dr. Arthur Ward of course are delighted to see the gamma system involved in models of why VL lesions do things to dyskinesias. But I seem to remember that his work with Jack Stern sort of came out the other way around. That is, when they stimulated in the VL, they produced inhibition of the gamma system and they thought that this was a disinhibition. Would you like to comment on that?

**Dr. Gilman:** Yes, I would like to comment on that. In 1960, Stern and Ward found that stimulation in the VL nucleus inhibited the afferent discharge of muscle spindles in the contralateral gastrocnemius-soleus muscle of pentobarbital-anesthetized cats. However, Yanagisawa, Narabayashi, and

Shimizu, in 1963, found that the effects of stimulating the VL nucleus are more complex than those reported by Stern and Ward. Under light anesthesia, high-frequency stimulation facilitated the responses of spindle afferents in extensor muscles; under moderate or deep anesthesia the responses were inhibited. The Yanagisawa group found the effects of stimulation to vary with the frequency of stimulation as well as with the depth of anesthesia. Furthermore, lesions of VL nucleus in experimental animals more closely replicate the studies in humans and our data appear to be more consistent when we produce lesions than the data resulting from stimulation experiments. It should be mentioned that our experiments showed an interesting elevation of spindle responses at temperatures between 0°C and − 10°C, a result that may be due to a stimulation effect or, more likely it may result from a decrease of the level of anesthesia.

**Dr. Cooper:** The cooling between zero and + 18 stimulates both centrally and peripherally and I think we reported that a long time ago. In fact the work was done here by Dr. Matsuoka. But even Hassler, whose work of course Morgenstern substantiated, has since come to a middle view that perhaps there is one kind of gamma fiber which is depressed and anolther which is not. So that we can compromise the situation there and call it a benign circle. Dr. Poirier, I'm sure, has a great deal to say about this because he has long been involved in the investigation of hypertonus from an anatomical and neurophysiological standpoint, and has been able to broaden his horizon and scope of investigation from anatomy to neurophysiology and neurochemistry. I have asked Dr. Poirier to act as our final discussant and to pull things together and attempt to resolve some of these problems that Dr. Gilman has raised.

**Dr. Poirier:** First I would like to extend my thanks on behalf of the group to Dr. Cooper and his staff for the opportunity we had to become so quickly acquainted with the pulvinar during this meeting.

I shall be informal and attempt to make a general summary instead of raising specific points which Dr. Gilman already did so well in reviewing the contribution of each speaker at this one day session. Therefore, I shall bring up only a few problems related to the various presentations. Clinically speaking, evidence was put forward suggesting that the pulvinar may play an important role in the control of language, and more especially in relation to anomia and aphasia. The pulvinar may also be involved in pain mechanisms and in the control of motor activity. This morning the anatomy of the pulvinar was well summarized. It was mentioned by Dr. Siqueira that it is especially related to the association cortex. On the other hand, Dr. Van Buren pointed out the observation that hypertrophy of the pulvinar is related to a greater development of the association cortex. As mentioned by Dr. Rakic, the pulvinar, during its development, receives some cells from the ganglionic eminence which gives rise to the basal ganglia. This appears to be an important point that needs to be clarified, possibly with histochemistry. Although we need more facts, it would be of interest to find out whether the pulvinar is in some way related to the basal ganglia as has been established for VL. It has been shown that the pulvinar is closely related to the cortex and more especially to the temporal lobe by numerous interconnecting fibers. Moreover, the pulvinar is crossed by important groups of fibers (cortico-tectal and cortico-tegmental) and we must take account of the latter fact when interpreting results derived from stimulation of the pulvinar.

In the light of these data it is difficult to choose which function among those mentioned today most particularly belongs to the pulvinar. I would be inclined to pick up the functions related to language. If I am correct, language disturbances have also been seen in association with temporal lobe lesions, and more specifically with those involving the temporal pole. Therefore, there is a functional relationship between the pulvinar and the temporal pole, the two being closely related by interconnecting nervous pathways. I think, however, that the anatomy of the topographical relationship between these structures has to be more precisely worked out using the silver impregnation technique for degenerating fibers from the cortex to the pulvinar and Nissl stain to disclose chromatolysis to detect the origin of the neurons from the pulvinar ending in the temporal lobe. This may also be clarified with·the neurophysiological approach.

Concerning the second point brought up by the clinicians in reference to the relief of spasticity by lesions in the pulvinar, it is difficult to identify the particular mechanism within the pulvinar that is responsible for such an effect. We, however, may recall in the light of this morning's reports and discussion of stimulation of the pulvinar that the latter structure is traversed by important fiber bundles which have their origins in the occipito-parietal and temporal cortices. Some of these fiber groups are certainly related to the control of eye movements. These different corticofugal fibers termed cortico-tectal and cortico-tegmental also reach the brain stem reticular formation. Does the interruption of latter groups of fibers at the level of pulvinar in patients have something to do with the reduction of spasticity? This hypothesis has to be supported by more experimental and clinical data.

The third point raised by our clinical colleagues concerns the mechanisms involved in the relief of pain associated with lesions of the pulvinar. I must say that I find it "painful" to explain these data in the light of our present knowledge of the pulvinar. In this case also we are dealing with nervous structures which constitute the pulvinar itself (such as the neurons themselves or fibers ending in the pulvinar), or else with fibers going through the pulvinar. In the light of the data presented today, I cannot offer any logical explanation of these observations pertaining to the relief of pain by pulvinectomy. I would like to complete this summary by comparing the VL and the pulvinar and pointing out the great amount of information which exists concerning the VL and its topographical relationship to tremor, rigidity or akinesia in comparison to our dearth of knowledge about the pulvinar at present. As shown on the first slide it has been established that the main outflow of the striopallidal system leaves the internal division of the pallidum and mainly reaches the VA-VL complex of the thalamus; but does not project to the pulvinar.

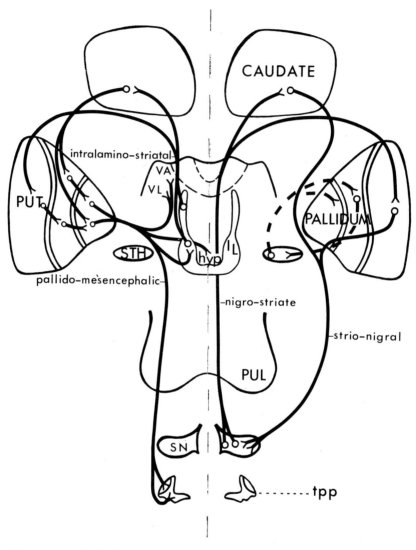

The striopallidal system includes, in addition to the caudate nucleus, putamen and pallidum, brain stem structures such as the intralaminar nuclei of the thalamus, the subthalamic nucleus and the substantia nigra which are interconnected with the striatum and pallidum through fibers which constitute loops within the striopallidal system. The second slide shows interconnecting fibers between VA and VL and the

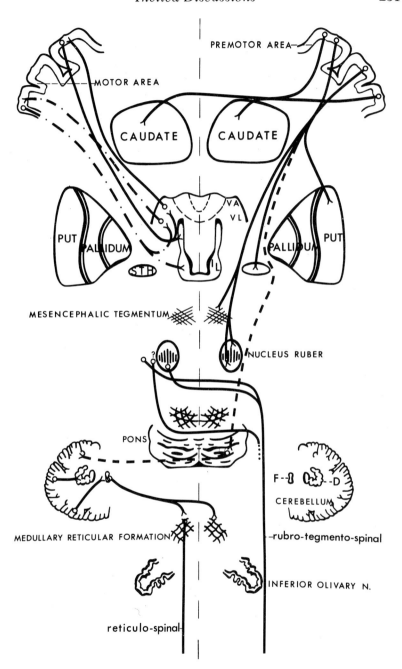

motor and premotor cortices which give rise to two groups of descending fibers: direct corticospinal and corticobulbar pathways and indirect cortico-subcortico-spinal pathways.

With the help of recently disclosed information concerning the extrapyramidal system we may now attempt a more logical explanation for the production and relief of rigidity, as mentioned by Dr. Gilman as for tremor and akinesia. As a matter of fact, a disturbance within this system, such as the loss of the dopaminergic mechanism for instance, leads to a functional imbalance within the neostriatum itself which, in turn, may affect the activity of the pallidum and, secondarily, the thalamus. As the latter structure through its VL and VA nuclei is related to the motor and premotor cortex, an impairment of the extrapyramidal system may finally lead to a disturbance in the alpha and gamma motoneurons. However, it now appears that the integrity of the gamma loop which is essential in the production of rigidity does not represent an important feature for the expression of tremor as the interruption of the gamma loop by sectioning the sensory spinal roots will not suppress postural tremor in patients and monkeys.

These and other data recently obtained with different approaches permit us to offer a more sound explanation of the mechanisms underlying rigidity, tremor, akinesia, dystonias, etc., and of their correction by surgery or other therapy. In reference to the pulvinar, however, we must confess that, except for the connections with the association cortex mentioned this morning we know very little about its whole nervous circuitry. It is expected that the clinical observation mentioned today regarding the stimulation and destruction of the pulvinar in man will attract the attention of research workers and stimulate them to gain as much information concerning the pulvinar as they have gained during the last decade for the VA and VL thalamic nuclei, research which was prompted by the disclosure of fascinating clinical data.

The reports of our clinical colleagues, I am sure, have convinced all of us that we must go back to work and learn much more about the pulvinar before we can attempt to determine its functions more precisely.

**EDITOR'S NOTE**

As a direct consequence of the symposium on the Pulvinar-LP Complex, a research affiliation was established between the Department of Neurologic Surgery at St. Barnabas Hospital and the Institute of Neurology and Psychiatry at Bucharest. The initial portion of this affiliation permitted Dr. Crighel of Bucharest to work at St. Barnabas Hospital for three months as a visiting scientist, with the specific goal of developing a systematic program of electrophysiological studies of the pulvinar in man, and the assessment of a group of patients before, during, and following cryopulvinectomy. The following paper summarizes preliminary findings in this program.

# CHAPTER 10

# PRELIMINARY ELECTROPHYSIOLOGICAL INVESTIGATIONS

# OF PULVINAR AND LP NUCLEUS IN MAN

E. CRIGHEL, I.S. COOPER, I. AMIN, J.M. WALTZ, AND J. ORZUCHOWSKI

GENERALLY, IN EXPERIMENTAL investigations in cat, the pulvinar-LP is considered as a functional complex involved in the transmission and processing of peripheral, especially visual, information (Buser, Borenstein, and Bruner, 1959; Crighel, 1972; Crighel and Kreindler, 1973; Godfrained, Meulders, and Veraart, 1972; Hotta and Kameda, 1963; Hotta and Terashima, 1966; Kreindler, Crighel, and Marinchescu, 1966; Kreindler, Crighel, and Marinchescu, 1968). The early appearance in phylogeny of the LP and the late appearance of Pul and the wide development of the pulvinar and its parallel evolution with the neocortex point to a differentiation in function of these two structures in higher mammals, and especially in man. One may presume that pulvinar assumes some integrative functions which LP had when it structurally prevailed. Therefore, in our investigations in man, reported in this preliminary paper, we were concerned especially with the study of the pulvinar. In some instances we have investigated the LP for comparison.

The investigations were performed as follows:

a. The changes of the spontaneous EEG and of flash (VER) or somesthetic (SER) evoked responses after a surgically produced cryolesion either only in Pul or combined with one in VL.

b. Responses evoked by peripheral stimuli (flash and somesthetic) in LP and Pul, cortical responses to LP or Pul electric stimulation, and the action of Pul tetanization on VER, were investigated during surgery.

This preliminary collaborative investigation has been concerned with only a few cases. Moreover, each patient, apart from the surgically produced lesion, had one or more prior lesions, due to his disease. Although there are many common findings regarding Pul or LP functions, the results are to be considered only as preliminary.

## A. Investigations Performed After Surgery

### 1. *The Spontaneous EEG*

The recordings were performed with a Grass EEG machine. The leads were mono- and bipolar; the electrodes were placed according to the 10–20 system.

The records after a pulvinar lesion generally, but not invariably, showed a worsening of the tracings, if changes in EEG existed before surgery, or the appearance of EEG changes if the traces were normal previous to surgery. The changes were characterized by theta or delta waves of high amplitude, isolated or in bursts. If such changes existed previously, these waves became higher and slower. The alterations were homolateral to the lesion and tended to be localized in fronto-temporal leads.

After 2 to 4 months the EEG tracings generally reverted to the initial preoperative pattern. In some cases they became normal, showing no differences between the two hemispheres, despite infliction of a lesion in ventrolateralis as well as pulvinar. In other cases the EEG changes have remained constant up to two years after cryopulvinectomy.

### 2. *Responses Evoked by Peripheral Stimuli Following a Pulvinar Lesion*

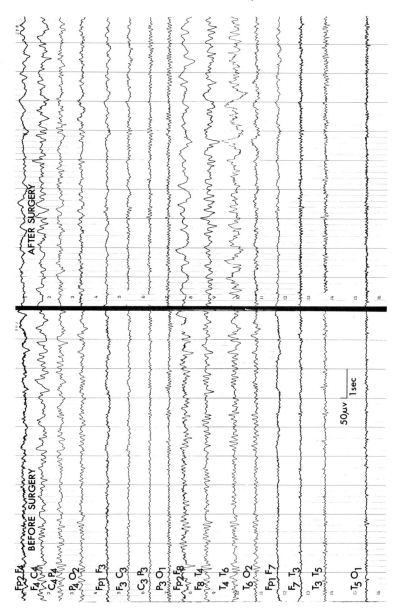

FIGURE 10–1. Patient with a right side caudate and internal capsule lesion. Theta and delta waves are seen on the right side, especially in temporal leads. After pulvinar cryolesion, note the worsening of the tracings.

a. Visual evoked responses (VER) were elicited by single bright flashes, delivered at random, at intervals varying from 2 to 4 seconds. The patient lay in a semi-obscure quiet room, the bulb of the stroboscope being situated 50 cm in front of his closed eyes. The responses, recorded by a GRASS oscillograph were averaged by a Mnemotron computer of average transients (CAT). The analysis duration was 500 ms. Twenty-five samples were averaged.

The VER in $P_z$ -$O_z$ started with a small negative wave and had a latency of 40 ms at the tip of this initial negativity. The succeeding waves were normal in amplitude and latency. After a latency of 150–175 ms an ample slow negative wave appeared. During natural sleep only a small long lasting negative wave with a latency of 100 ms was seen. Awakening after sleep this slow late wave disappeared.

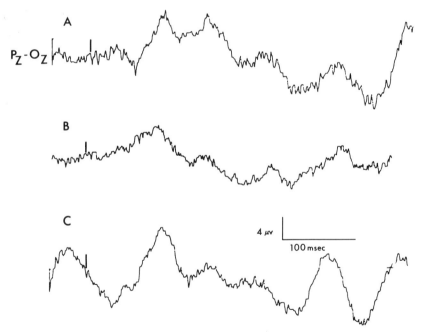

FIGURE 10–2. VER in a patient following left pulvinar and VL lesion. A. Patient awake; note the late, ample, negative, slow wave. B. Same patient during sleep; only a small long lasting negative wave is seen. C. Same patient awakening; note the disappearance of the late negative wave. General legend:in all figures the bars indicate the moment of flash delivery.

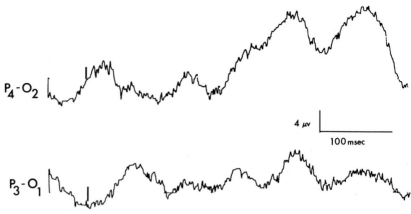

FIGURE 10–3. The same patient as in Fig. 2. VER recorded from parieto-occipital leads. Note the late, slow, negative wave in the side contralateral to the lesion.

In parieto-occipital leads ($P_4$-$O_2$ resp. $P_3$-$O_1$) the late ample negative wave appeared only contralateral to the lesion.
In a case with a large caudate and capsular lesion prior to surgery, a late ample negative VER was found before surgery, homolateral to the lesion. It remained unchanged following cryopulvinectomy.

b. Somesthetic evoked responses (SER) were elicited by single electric shocks of 0.5 msec duration on the palmar surface of the middle finger. The responses were recorded in C-P leads (resp. $C_4$-$P_4$ and $C_3$-$P_3$) homolaterally and contralaterally to the finger stimulation. The averaging was performed as in VER.

The SER showed also the appearance of a late negative slow wave contralateral to the pulvinar lesion. It was not so evident as in the case of the VER.

It should be noted that averaging the basic EEG activity for the same period of analysis and also 25 samples showed a tendency for higher synchronizing contralaterally to the lesion.

## B. Investigations Performed During Surgery

1. Responses in Pul-LP were evoked by peripheral stimuli (bright flashes) and electric shocks on the contralateral and homolateral medial finger. The responses were recorded bipolarly by means of a coaxial electrode; the distance between the noninsulated tip of the central wire and the

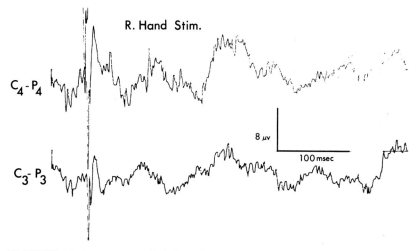

R. Hand Stim.

C₄-P₄

C₃-P₃

8 μv

100 msec

FIGURE 10–4. Patient with left pulvinar lesion. SER in $C_4$-$P_4$ and $C_3$-$P_3$ leads. The late, slow, negative wave (less marked than in VER), is also seen contralateral to the pulvinar lesion.

noninsulated ring of the steel tube was 1 mm; the electrode was introduced stereotaxically to the target (LP and then in Pul) and checked by X-ray.

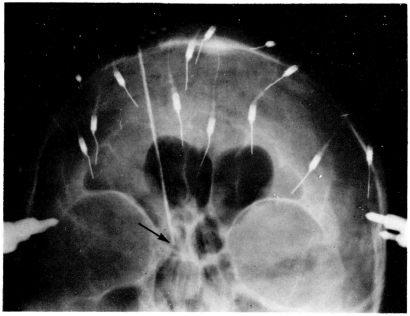

FIGURE 10–5A. A-P and lateral roentgenogram, to confirm the depth electrode location.

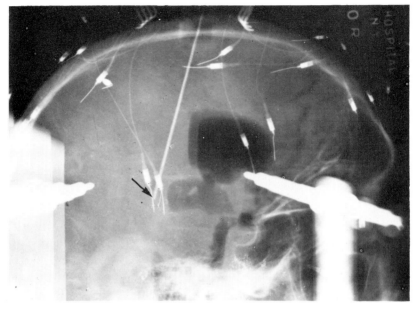

Figure 10–5B

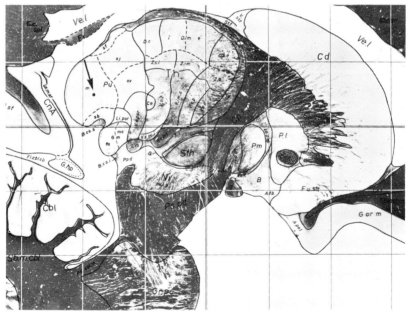

Figure 10–5C

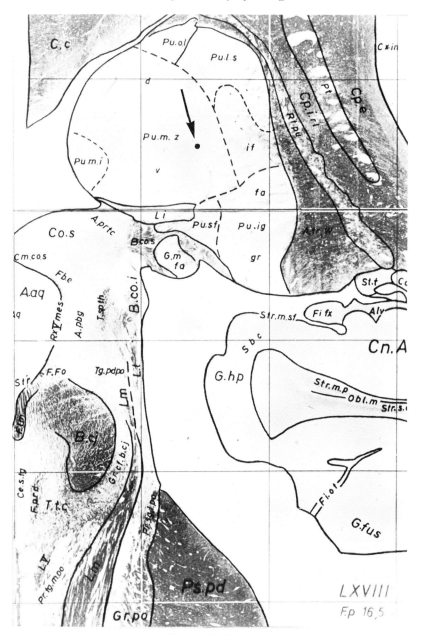

Figure 10–5D

In LP no responses to flash or to somesthetic stimuli were found.

In pulvinar a point was found in which only responses to flashes were seen. The response had a latency of 50 ms and showed only a split negative slow wave.

**R. Pul. VER**

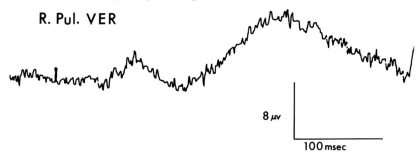

8 µv

100 msec

**R Pul. L. Finger Stim.**

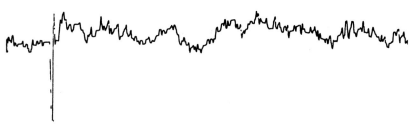

FIGURE 10–6. Patient with left hemiplegia, hypertonia and athetotic movements. A. Responses to flashes (VER) in right (R) pulvinar (Pul). B. No responses to left hand stimulation.

Another point in another patient showed a very ample response to flash with an initial split positivity, followed by a high negative-positive wave. The latency of the initial positivity was 40 ms.

There was also an ample response only to contralateral finger stimulation with the recording electrode in the same point. This response consisted of an initial positive phase with 30 ms latency, followed by an ample negative-positive wave.

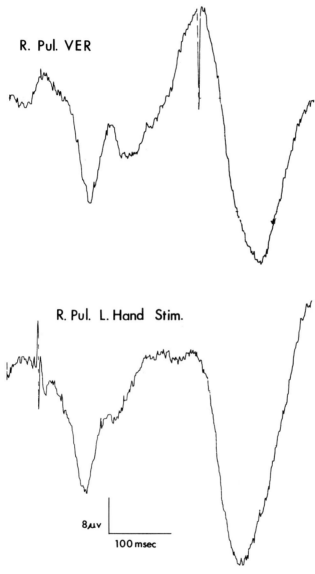

**R. Pul. VER**

**R. Pul. L. Hand Stim.**

8 μv

100 msec

FIGURE 10–7. Patient with right caudate and internal capsule lesion. Left hemiplegia and hypertonia. A. Responses to flashes in right (R) pulvinar (Pul). B. Responses to left hand stimulation.

The spontaneous activity in Pul showed waves of 5–6 c/s, small or ample, continuous or in bursts. It should be noted that the same type of waves were often found in the homolateral anterior temporal or temporo-frontal leads.

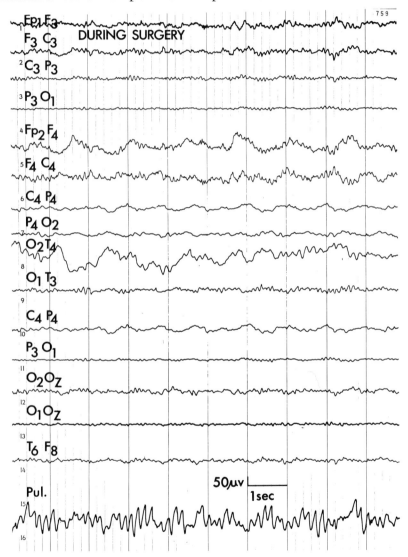

FIGURE 10–8. The same patient as in Fig. 7. Spontaneous EEG and spontaneous activity in right pulvinar. Note that the same type of waves are seen in the homolateral anterior temporal leads, as in right pulvinar.

## 3. Stimulation of the Pul-LP Complex

No neocortical response could be elicited by the stimulation of the LP points investigated, by single pulses or with a rate of 8–10 c/s, with rectangular pulses of 0.5 ms duration and until 3–4 mA, in contrast with earlier experience reported in this symposium, in which higher voltage stimulation was employed.

Repetitive stimulation with 8–10 c/s elicited in a patient a very long lasting myoclonus, contralateral to the LP stimulated in both arm and leg. In the same patient, who had a spastic hemiplegia, stroke of the paralyzed arm or foot, or other peripheral stimuli, also elicited a very intense clonic discharge.

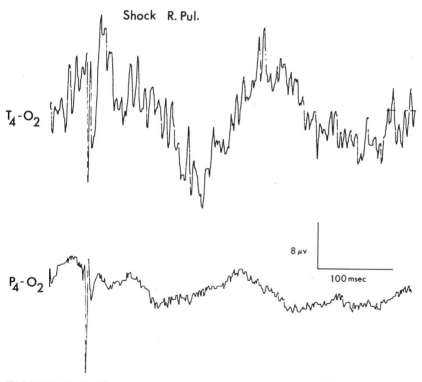

FIGURE 10–9. The same patient as shown in Fig. 6, following single shocks to right pulvinar. Responses are seen in parieto-occipital and temporo-occipital leads, homolateral to the stimulated pulvinar.

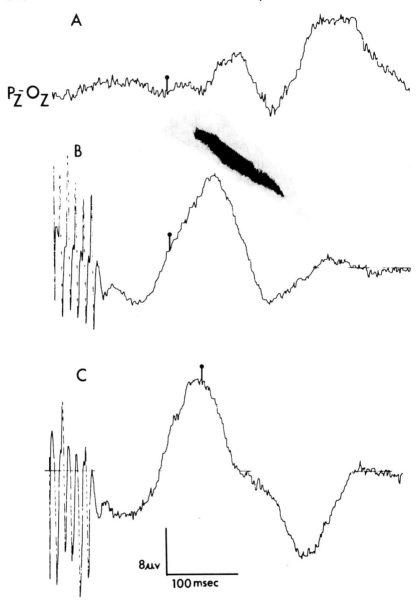

FIGURE 10–10. The same patient as shown in Figs. 6 and 9. Pulvinar tetanization, 100 c/s, 2 mA, 0.5 msec each stimulus, 50 msec duration of the train, enhanced the positive phases of the VER. A. Control; B. 100 msec delay between the end of the tetanization and the flash; C. 150 msec delay.

Single shocks of lower intensity in Pul elicited homolateral neocortical responses. The responses were primarily parieto-occipital. They were positive-negative responses of various amplitude and had a long latency of 70–80 ms.

Tetanization of the same point in Pul with 100 c/s and 50 ms duration of the train of stimuli modifies the reactivity of the visual area to peripheral stimuli. When such tetanization preceded the flash by 100–150 ms it depressed the negative and enhanced the positive early components of the VER.

## DISCUSSION

The data from the present collaboration study, actually carried out six months after this symposium, are in accordance with many of the electro-physiological data presented earlier by Cooper *et al.* (Cooper, Amin, Chandra, and Waltz, 1972). Our findings concerning the role of the medial nucleus of pulvinar in man in reception of information from the periphery and their transmission to the neocortex are analogous with those found by other authors in their experimental studies on lateralis posterior nucleus of cat thalamus (Buser, Borenstein, and Bruner, 1959; Crighel, 1972; Hotta and Terashima, 1966; Kreindler, Crighel, and Marinchescu, 1966; Kreindler, Crighel, and Marinchescu, 1968). The pulvinar in man has demonstrated the same type of neuronal pools as the LP in cat; that is, both monosensorial and polysensorial points (Hotta and Kameda, 1963; Kreindler, Crighel, and Marinchescu, 1966). We also found a commutation (switching) function with the projection of these points in temporal and parietal areas (Kreindler, Crighel, and Marinchescu, 1968). The differences in latency, pattern, and amplitude found in different patients may depend in each case on a previous surgical lesion or the pathology underlying the patient's disease.

This study has also demonstrated that pulvinar tetanization modifies the reactivity of the visual area to peripheral stimuli, similar to that previously observed following tetanization of the cat LP (Battersby and Oestereich, 1963; Brown and Marco, 1967; Crighel and Kreindler, 1973).

In one patient with spasticity, the LP stimulation elicited clonic movements in the spastic limbs like those elicited by a peripheral stimulus. It is assumed that in both cases the same mechanism was involved; that is, a dysfunction in the synchronization of the sensorial input and the motor organization at the thalamo-cortical level. The same phenomenon was not seen when pulvinar was stimulated in the same patient. This suggests that in man LP is more related to motor organization, while pulvinar is more directly concerned with the processing of information from the periphery.

Our data demonstrate that Pul projects on the neocortex not only in the anterior temporal area (Siqueira and Franks, 1973), but also the parietal area (Van Buren, 1973). In this particular study we did not find a contralateral projection of the points investigated in Pul. This possibility is not excluded because even in cat not all the points from the Pul-LP complex project contralaterally (Crighel and Kreindler, 1973; Kreindler, Crighel, and Marinchescu, 1968). Moreover, the earlier studies of Cooper *et al.* (Cooper, Amin, Chandra, and Waltz, 1973) suggest such a projection.

It is difficult to explain the appearance of a long lasting slow activity in the homolateral neocortex, especially in the temporo-frontal leads after cryogenic pulvinar lesions. The EEG changes tend to occur in the same area where Pul presumably projects.

It is even more difficult to explain the appearance of a late slow wave appearing in VER and SER. In VER this wave appears especially in midline record and contralateral to the Pul lesion. The same type of VER was seen in patients with other thalamic and brain stem lesions (Crighel and Poilici, 1968). The disappearance of this late slow component of the VER during the period of awakening of one patient points to a functional disturbance produced by the Pul lesion, resembling that produced by phenobarbitone on brain stem synchronizing structures (Crighel and Poilici, 1968). This is similar to other findings (Cooper, Amin, Chandra, and Waltz, 1973) which showed the occasional lessening of hyperactivity and epileptiform EEG activity in some patients after cryopulvinectomy.

In conclusion, it seems that Pul in man has a very complex function and presumes some functions which are performed by LP in cat in which Pul is a rudimentary structure.

## References

Battersby, W.G. and Oestereich, R.E.: Neural limitations of visual excitability. IV. Photic enhancement following lateral thalámic stimulation. *Electroencph. Clin. Neurophysiol. 15*:849–863, 1963.

Brown, T.S. and Marco, L.A.: Effects of stimulation of the superior colliculus and lateral thalamus on visual evoked responses. *Electroenceph. Clin. Neurophysiol. 22*:150–158, 1967.

Buser, P., Borenstein, P., and Bruner, J.: Etude des systemes associatifs visuels et auditifs chez le chat anesthesie au chloralose. *Electroenceph. Clin. Neurophysiol. 11*:305–324, 1959.

Cooper, I.S., Amin, I., Chandra, R., and Waltz, J.M.: A surgical investigation of the clinical physiology of the LP-Pulvinar complex in man. *J. Neurol. Sci., 18*:89–110, 1973.

Cooper, I.S., Amin, I., Chandra, R., and Waltz, J.M.: Clinical Physiology of Motor Contributions of the Pulvinar in Man: A Study of Cryopulvinectomy. In I.S. Cooper, M. Riklan and P. Rakic (Eds.), *The Pulvinar-LP Complex*. Springfield, Charles C Thomas, 1974.

Crighel, E.: Integration functions and information processing at the thalamocortical level. *Rev. Roum. Neurol. 9*:(1972) in press.

Crighel, E. and Poilici, T.: Photic evoked responses in patients with thalamic and brain stem lesions. *Conf. Neurol.* (Basel) *30*:301–312, 1968.

Crighel, E. and Kreindler, A.: The role of the thalamic Pulvinar-lateralis posterior complex in modulating neocortical reactivity. In I.S. Cooper, M. Riklan, and P. Rakic (Eds.) *The Pulvinar-LP Complex*. Springfield: Charles C Thomas, 1974.

Godfrained, J.M., Meulders, M., and Veraart, C.: Visual properties of neurons in pulvinar nucleus lateralis posterior and nucleus suprageniculatus thalami in the cat. I. Qualitative investigation. *Brain Research, 44*:403–526, 1972.

Hotta, T. and Kameda, K.: Interactions between somatic and visual or auditory responses in the thalamus of the cat. *Exp. Neurol. 8*:1–13, 1963.

Hotta, T. and Terashima, S.: Correlations between activity of the visual cortex and the somato-visual interaction in the lateral thalamus of cats. *Brain Research, 2*:160–172, 1966.

Kreindler, A., Crighel, E., and Marinchescu, C.: Neocortical excitability and relationships with the pulvinar-lateralis posterior complex. In D. Gonzalez Martin (Ed.), *Cortico-Subcortical Relationships in Sensory Regulation*. Havana, Acad. Sci., pp. 75–84, 1966.

Kreindler, A., Crighel, E., and Marinchescu, C.: Integrative activity of the thalamic pulvinar-lateralis posterior complex and interrelations with the neocortex. *Exp. Neurol. 22*:423–435, 1968.

Siqueira, E.B. and Franks, L.: Anatomic connections of the pulvinar. In I.S. Cooper, M. Riklan, and P. Rakic (Eds.), *The Pulvinar-LP Complex.* Springfield, Charles C Thomas, 1974.

Van Buren, J.M.: Invited Discussion. In I.S. Cooper, M. Riklan, and P. Rakic (Eds.), *The Pulvinar-LP Complex.* Springfield, Charles C Thomas, 1974.

## LIST OF ILLUSTRATIONS

276

## LIST OF TABLES

# NAME INDEX

Adachi, K., 133
Aikawa, S., 141, 170, 201, 202, 213, 231
Ainsworth, A., 78, 79, 118, 128, 132
Akert, K., 118, 122, 133
Albe-Fessard, E., 36, 51, 96, 118, 131, 227, 230
Alberts, W.W., 132
Aleonard, P., 118, 131
Allan, C.M., 162, 169
Altman, J., 20, 27
Amin, I., 118, 132, 143, 169, 202, 231, 267, 268, 269
Andersen, P., 78, 96, 120, 128, 132, 136
Anderson, F.D., 113, 120, 135
Andersson, S.A., 78, 120, 128, 132, 134, 135
Andy, O.J., 140, 160, 170
Angevine, J.B., 20, 24, 27
Arfel, G., 51, 118, 131
Armengol, V., 52, 61, 92

Bailey, P., 119, 133, 220, 231
Barlone, M., 93
Battersby, W.G., 81, 92, 94, 267, 269
Berry, C.M., 96, 113
Bertrand, G., 119, 132
Bignal, K.E., 92
Bishop, G.H., 110, 113
Bisiach, E., 190, 191
Blick, K.I., 170, 180, 183
Boggen, R.H., 200, 231
Borenstein, P., 92, 254, 267, 269
Borke, R.C., 67, 76, 140, 182, 184, 201, 232
Boulder Committee, 13, 23, 27
Boyd, J.D., 13, 28
Brissaud, E., 36, 51
Brown, J.W., 141, 142, 157, 165, 166, 167, 169, 186, 191, 220, 230
Brown, T.S., 81, 90, 92, 94, 118, 131, 267, 269
Bruner, J., 92, 254, 267, 269

Buser, P., 80, 92, 254, 267, 269

Campus-Ortega, J.A., 52, 61, 78, 79, 132
Carpenter, M., 140, 171, 235
Chandra, R., 267, 268, 269
Chow, K.L., 37, 51, 118, 128, 200, 231
Ciemens, V., 182, 183
Clark, W.E.L., 10, 27, 140, 169
Clüver, P.F. de V., 52, 61, 79, 132
Cohen, B., 58, 59, 61
Collins, W.F., 99, 101, 114
Cooper, I.S., 36, 51, 52, 60, 139, 141, 142, 143, 157, 161, 162, 163, 165, 167, 169, 171, 191, 202, 221, 230, 231, 267, 268, 269
Copack, P., 244
Cowey, A., 129, 132
Cragg, B.G., 78, 79, 118, 128, 132, 133
Crighel, E., 91, 92, 94, 130, 135, 137, 140, 166, 169, 170, 202, 227, 231, 254, 267, 268, 269
Crosby, E.C., 93
Crouch, R.L., 37, 51

Daroff, R., 136
Davies, T.L., 29
Déjerine, J., 36, 51
Dekaban, A., 6, 7, 12, 27
DeLaherran, J., 118, 131
DeLattre, L.D., 132
Derome, P., 51, 118, 131
Dewulf, A., 21, 27
Diller, L., 160, 163, 171

Eisenson, J., 163, 169
Essick, C.R., 18, 23, 27

Fedio, P., 51, 170, 173, 174, 176, 177, 178, 180, 182, 183, 201, 231
Feferman, M.D., 96, 113
Feinstein, B., 132
Feldman, M.H., 58, 61

278

# SUBJECT INDEX

## A

Air ventriculography, 203
Alpha appearance, 121–127
  EEG activation, 127
  EOG alterations, 127
Alpha block, 133–134
Alpha motoneurons,
  disturbance in, 252
Alpha rhythm, pulvinar (*see* Pulvinar)
Alpha rhythm appearance, 120–133
  cortical and pulvinar, 120–133
    during eye closure, 122
    during fixation-holding, 123
    during information processing, 133
    during pulvinar stimulation, 124, 130
    during rest, 120
    during saccadic eye movement, 124
    "isolated thalamic alpha", 121, 128
Alpha rhythm generation, 130
Amygdala, 32, 52
  cell origin, 32
  connections, 52
Anesthesia, level of, 247
Anomia, definition, 164, 175
  frequency, 176
  location, 177
  occurrence, 176, 191
  retrieval deficit, 181
  site of, 176
  threshold, 177–178
  transient, 181
Anomic response, definition, 186, 192, 238
  language disturbance, 238
  prolonged aphasia, 238
Anomics, cortical, 190
Ansa lenticularis, 59
Aphasia, definition, 184
  demonstration, 184–185
    object naming, 184–185

Aphasia, prolonged, 182, 238
  anomic response, 238
Aphasia tests, 163–164
Aphasic patients, classification, 190
Aphasic response, 185
  caudate stimulation, 185
  pulvinar stimulation, 185
  performance tests, 185
Arrest response, definition, 185, 238
Arteriotomy, femoral, cats, 97
Association cortex, development, 65
  expansion, 76
  in man, in monkey, 76
Association neocortex, location, 4
Association nuclei, 24
Augmenting responses, 193
Axons, activation, 62
  afferent, ingrowth of, 10
  convergence, 66

## B

Basal ganglia, anlage of, 13
  ganglionic eminence, 12–13
  development, 233, 248
  neurons, origin of, 26, 31
  telencephalon, primordial source for, 33
Basal ganglia surgery, effects on speech, 161
Beckman DC Electrodes (*see* Electrodes)
Behavior, thalamocortical systems in, 168
  participation of, 168
Behavior, integrated, 139
  neural factors, 139
Behavioral changes, after pulvinar surgery, 222
Bender-Gestalt test, performance scores, 155
  basis of, 155

282

## V

## W

## Z